The Complete Guide to Foot Reflexology

(Third Edition)

Barbara
and
Kevin
Kunz

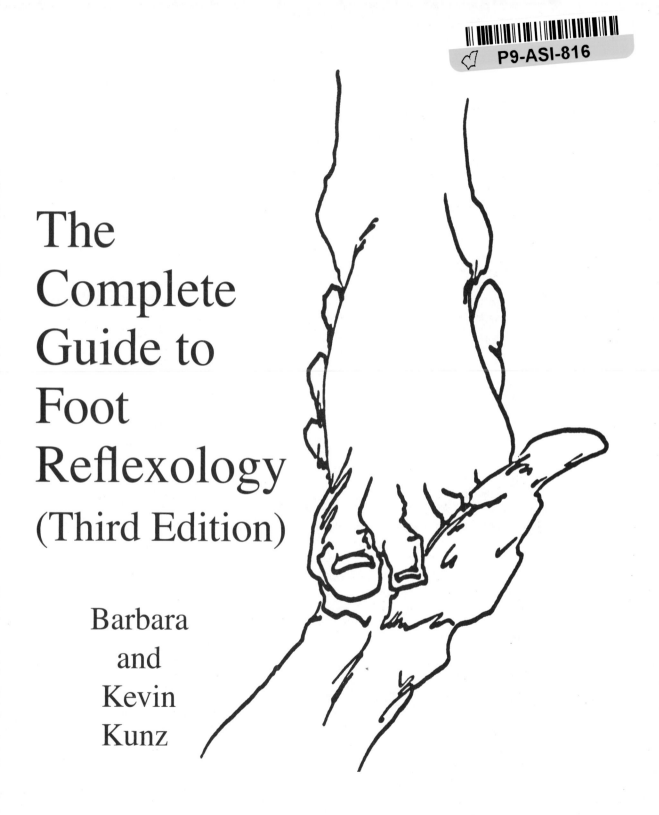

Books by Barbara and Kevin Kunz
The Complete Guide to Foot Reflexology, 1980
Hand and Foot Reflexology, A Self- Help Guide, Simon & Schuster, 1984
Hand Reflexology Workbook, Prentice Hall, 1985
The Practitioner's Guide to Reflexology, Prentice Hall, 1985
The Complete Guide to Foot Reflexology (Revised), RRP Press,1993
The Parent's Guide to Reflexology, Random House, 1995
Hand Reflexology Workbook (Revised), RRP Press, 1999
Medical Applications of Reflexology, RRP Press,1999
My Reflexologist Says Feet Don't Lie, RRP Press, 2001
Reflexology, Health at your fingertips, Dorling Kindersly, 2003

Kunz and Kunz titles are published in twelve languages and 30 foreign language editions. Reflexology training materials are available. For more information, see www.reflexology-research.com.

Published by RRP Press
P. O. Box 35820, Albuquerque, NM 87176
Phone 505-344-9392, FAX 505-344-0246, E-mail footc@mac.com
Web pages: www.reflexology-research.com, www.foot-reflexologist.com, www.myreflexologist.com

Reflexology is not intended to be a substitute for medical care. If you have a health problem, consult a medical professional.

10 9 8 7 6 5 4 3 2 1

Illustrations and book design by Barbara Kunz
Cover and chapter divider art by Camille Young

ISBN 0-9606070-1-3

Table of Contents

Index

Introduction

"I've never met this man before and he knows all about me!" The scene was a reflexology demonstration at a San Francisco health food store. I had just picked up the woman's foot and asked her, "Do you have hearing problems?" She responded that, even at her young age, she was hard of hearing. She walked around after my session repeating her amazement to any and all.

And then there was reaction at another demonstration. I looked at the woman's foot and commented, "I've worked on these feet before." She was very surprised. I had worked on her feet once and it was ten years before.

The insights reflected in these stories resulted from years of work at identifying a reflexology assessment and relating it to a client. Being a complete reflexologist is not only about good technique application, it's also about being knowledgeable, systematic, and capable of reading stress patterns and relating them to a client and / or a health professional.

This book is about taking a systematic approach to reflexology work. The future of reflexology lies not only in its effectiveness but also in the ability of its practitioners to communicate that effectiveness in a comprehendible and measurable manner.

With this, the third edition of *The Complete Guide to Foot Reflexology*, our goal is to give you the tools you need to make you The Complete Reflexologist. This edition details reflexology work as quantifiable and gives you the skills you need as a successful practitioner, business person, and professional.

"Knowing all about" someone from his or her feet is not an isolated, random event. The ability to match stress cues in the feet to real life health situations is a skill delineated in this text. Both clientele and medical professionals respond to a chronicling of: (1) standardized technique procedures for assessment using cues and inferences, (2) research indicating possibilities of results for clientele as well as defining reflexology's role in evidence-based medicine, and (3) photographic documentation of reflexology work.

Translating more than thirty years of reflexology experiences into a systematic approach to reflexology knowledge has created an endlessly interesting process for us. It has resulted in eight books translated into multiple languages and foreign editions, more than a hundred newsletter issues, and copious material on the Internet. (www.reflexology-research.com, www.foot-reflexologist.com, www.myreflexologist.com).

Over the years we've tackled our concerns about reflexology, working toward the continuation of the idea and the success of its practitioners. This has included:

• putting into written form the verbal tradition of reflexology (the original *The Complete Guide to Foot Reflexology*);

• describing a theory of reflexology grounded in the nervous system, developing assessment in observation of stress cues and drawing inferences and working to create professionalism in reflexology (*The Complete Guide to Foot Reflexology (Revised)*;

• working to secure the legal right to practice in the United States (noted at www.foot-reflexologist.com);

• elucidating and making known the available research (www.reflexology-research.com);

• expanding reflexology work to include self-help reflexology applications (*Hand and Foot Reflexology, A self-help guide*, and *Reflexology, Health at your fingertips*, and

• creating a quantifiable approach to hand reflexology (*Hand Reflexology Workbook*).

As you read and study this book, keep in mind that the future of reflexology is, quite literally, in your hands. We encourage you to contribute your own discoveries and to join the effort to place reflexology in the vanguard of health practices.

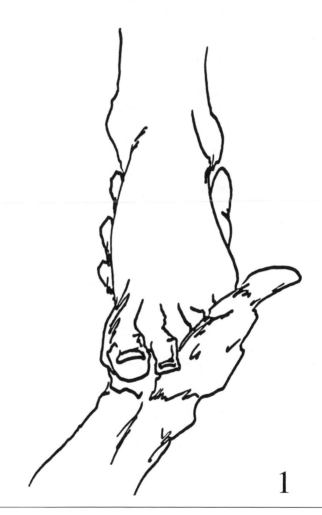

1

The Theory of Reflexology

The Theory of Reflexology

Any field of study has premises whose purpose is to tie it together into a coherent whole. Reflexology too has principles that serve to unify it as an integrated system. These principles, although simple, make a profound statement about the body and its functions. Foot reflexology is the study and practice of working reflexes in the feet that correspond to other parts of the body. With specific hand and finger techniques, reflexology provides stimulation and, thus, causes responses (relaxation) in corresponding parts of the body. Relaxation is the first step to the body's return to a state of equilibrium, or homeostasis, in which circulation can flow unimpeded to supply nutrients and oxygen to the cells. Research has demonstrated such change resulting from reflexology work. A change of blood flow to the kidneys was shown before and after reflexology work.[1] Improvement in blood flow to the intestines was also demonstrated.[2] With the restoration of homeostasis, the body's organs and muscles, which are actually aggregations of cells, may then return to a normal state of function as well.

One's state of health depends on this ability to rebound to homeostasis after a trauma or injury (i. e., injury, disease, stress). So we can say it is the very purpose of reflexology to trigger this return. Since stress and disease are ongoing facts of life for most of us, reflexology, in addition to its therapeutic uses, can serve as a preventive program. It enables each individual, on a daily basis, to help his or her body restore and maintain its natural state of homeostasis.

The reflexes in the feet are actually "reflections" of body parts. Their locations and relationships to each other on the feet follow a logical anatomical pattern which closely resembles that of the body itself. The premise of how the reflexes of the feet correspond to the anatomy of the whole body is simple: the actual physical image of the body is projected onto them. This image is organized with the use of zone theory.

It may be that stress is the single greatest threat to the body's equilibrium. Research of the last twelve years has created a more complete image of the impact of reflexology work on the body's stress pattern. Foot reflexology is now seen as the study and practice of applying pressure techniques to

[1] Sudmeier, I., Bodner, G., Egger, I., Mur, E., Ulmer, H. and Herold, M. (Universitatsklinik fur Innere Medizin, Inssbruk, Austria) "Anderung der nierendurchblutung durch organassoziierte reflexzontherapie am fuss gemussen mit farbkodierter doppler-sonograhpie," Forsch Komplementarmed 1999, Jum;6(3):129-34

[2] J, Egger I, Bodner G, Eibl G, Hartig F, Pfeiffer KP, Herold M., "Influence of reflex zone therapy of the feet on intestinal blood flow measured by color Doppler sonography," [Article in German] Forsch Komplementarmed Klass Naturheilkd. 2001 Apr;8(2):86-9

pressure sensors in the feet. These pressure techniques serve to relax pressure sensors in the feet (foot stress), to interrupt stress patterns between various body parts (reflex stress), and to trigger a relaxation response throughout the body (body stress).

The feet are a part of the body's overall response to stress. Reflex areas reflect the overall dynamic state of tension that exists between all body parts. Observable cues such as puffiness indicate that stress has occurred and the body is adapting to it. The individual's foot reflex areas reflect the individual's overall state of tension that has resulted from a lifetime of adaptation to stress. Stress cues in the feet are a roadmap to the reflexologist. Wherever it is found on a foot, it is a sign that stress and its effect have begun to accumulate in the corresponding parts of the body. The reflexologist observes the cues of stress and applies pressure techniques to relax the indicated stresses. The goal of the reflexologist is to create a relaxation response keyed to the individual and his or her stress. The result of such work has been defined by research as impacting health and well-being.

Reflexology Defined by Research

Major research findings show that reflexology: impacts disease, improves quality of life, and influences the workings of the body. Not only has the research pointed to plausible explanations for how reflexology works, but the studies have also demonstrated an instrumental role for reflexology in a modern medical system.

Among some forty-five controlled studies, reflexology is shown to have impact in the treatment of disease. Reflexology work was found to be effective in impacting disorders such as diabetes, constipation, headache, low white blood cell count, multiple sclerosis, and dyspepsia as well as symptoms of high cholesterol and coronary heart disease.

Quality of life improvements were seen in studies involving reflexology work and individuals of all ages. Studies with children showed improved control over encopresis (fecal incontinence). For women, birthing was shown to be easier following reflexology work as well as improved lactation. Symptoms of menopause, premenstrual syndrome and amenorrhea were impacted positively. Post-surgical pain and the pain following lithotrity (recovery from kidney stone surgery) was lessened.

Research showed that "...older adults (who walked on a reflexology mat of imitation cobblestones) experienced significant improvements in mental and physical well-being, including reductions in blood pressure and pain levels. … Elderly participants in the study experienced considerable improvements in their ability to perform 'activities of daily living,' increased psychosocial well-being, and significantly reduced daytime sleepiness and pain. Participants also reported greatly improved perceptions of control over falls and had reductions in resting diastolic blood pressure."[1]

For cancer patients, quality of life improvements following reflexology work were wide-ranging. In one study of cancer patients, "100% of the reflexology group benefited from an improvement in quality of life: appearance, appetite, breathing, communication (doctors), communication (family), communication (nurses), concentration, constipation, diarrhoea, fear of future, isolation, micturition, mobility, mood, nausea, pain, sleep and tiredness."[2] Another study of cancer patients showed a significant decrease in pain and anxiety with the authors noting "This has important implications for nursing practice as both professionals and lay people can be taught reflexology. Reflexology is a simple technique for human touch which can be performed anywhere, requires no special equipment, is non-invasive and does not interfere with patients' privacy." [3]

Studies show the specific impact of reflexology's influence on the body and clarify how reflexology works. Research demonstrated changes in measurable aspects of the body's functioning: free radicals in the blood, blood sugar levels, heart mechanisms, blood flow to the kidneys and blood flow to the intestines. Research defines reflexology's role as a complement to medicine and an enhancement to quality of life.

Reflexology Defined

Reflexology is the physical act of applying pressure to the feet with specific thumb, finger, and hand techniques without the use of oil or lotion based on a system of zones and areas that reflect an image of the body on the feet, with a premise that such work effects a physical change in the body. (Kunz and Kunz, *Reflexions*, Nov. / Dec. 1983)

[1] Fuzhong Li, Peter Harmer, Nicole L. Wilson, K. John Fisher, "Healthy Benefits of Cobblestone-Mat Walking: Preliminary Findings," *Journal of Aging and Physical Activity*, 11(4), October 2003, p. 1

[2] Hodgson, H. "Does reflexology impact on cancer patients' quality of life?," *Nursing Standard*, 14, 31, pp. 33-38

[3] Stephenson, N. L., Weinrich, S. P. and Tavakoli, A. S., "The effects of foot reflexology on anxiety and pain in patients with breast and lung cancer," *OncolNursForum* 2000, Jan.-Feb.;27(1):67-72

Man's stride in walking sets him off from other creatures on earth. The elements of the foot as an educable sensory organ provide its ability to function for locomotion. This view suggests that the foot contributes to two basic integrated functions of the body, the stride mechanism and the survival mechanism. The foot is thus a participant in the body's interactions with both the internal and the external worlds.

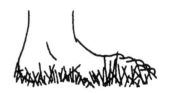

Adulthood and civilization join to create a lessened sensory demand on the feet and the body as a whole. Civilization has given us shoes to walk in and smooth surfaces to walk on. The foot no longer has practice at traversing rough terrain. Adulthood encourages routine, a kind of "sameness" of sensory experience. The routine, for example, of going to work and working at the same time, in the same place, at the same job creates a sameness of sensory information. Wear and tear is the result of repetitive, uninterrupted demands on the body.

It is the role of the foot in walking that provides the reflexologist with the opportunity to, literally, step in and interrupt stress. The foot is a sensory organ. It specializes in gathering information that makes locomotion possible. By sensing pressure, stretch, and movement, the foot contributes to the overall functioning of the body. The reflexologist, through the application of pressure techniques, interrupts the stress experienced by the foot and the whole body in moving about.

The stimulus of pressure prompts the body to respond in a predictable manner. The application of pressure techniques to particular parts of the foot by the reflexologist creates a stimulus to which the body must respond. The response of the body is predictable within the functions of the nervous system. Reflexology can be defined by the basic body mechanisms whose stress it interrupts.

Foot Stress

It is a commonly voiced truism that there are five senses: sight, hearing, touch, taste, and smell. But these five senses would be unable to explore the world around us were it not for our other "senses" - those that make movement possible. Pressure, stretch, and movement are the senses that provide us with the means to move about and interact with the external world.

The foot is a specialist in gathering pressure, stretch, and movement information. This information is necessary to create the purposeful activity of walking. To participate in such activity, the foot maintains a level of tension, or foot stress. A level of stress is needed so that each foot step is not a new

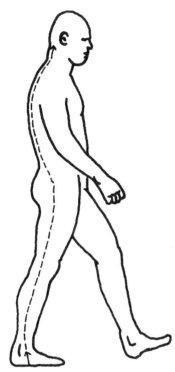

Feedback: Information gathered from pressure sensors in the foot is relayed to the brain.

undertaking. A preset level of instructions makes walking or any other activity smooth and continuous.

Pressure

Proprioception is a type of sensation from muscles, joints, and so on that conveys information about their relationship to the rest of the body so that posture is maintained by reflex movement. Of particular importance is deep pressure from the bottoms of the feet.

To move, the body must see itself. Such perception requires information about muscles, joints, and tendons. Sophisticated gauges in the muscles, tendons, and joints measure the pressure, stretch, and movement experienced by each. From such information, the body creates a picture of itself. Proprioception is the name given to such sensory perception. Proprioception means, literally, "to perceive oneself." Proprioceptors measure the foot's activities. They report on whether the foot is standing or sitting, walking or running, encased in a shoe or bare.

The foot is a sensory organ whose pressure sensors provide key information about body position. The foot, thus, acts as a means of receiving feedback about the external environment. Such feedback shapes our movements. Each stimulus is responded to accordingly. A rock underfoot calls for a different response than a sharp object underfoot. An image of what is underfoot is a means to survival. Without this feedback injury may occur that could have been avoided.

Stride

The gathering of sensory information by the foot is conducted for a purpose: the purpose of locomotion. To make locomotion possible, muscle groups throughout the body respond in sequence. The stage of the sequence is signaled by a particular sensory event: the pressure of the surface being walked on, the stretch of muscle in response to the surface, and the speed at which the surface is encountered. The net result is the coordinated activity of walking.

Organized activity such as walking requires direction from the brain. Every day is not a new day for the foot or any other sensory organ. Using information gathered over a lifetime, instructions are preprogrammed in anticipation of events to come, such as standing or walking. When the appropriate stimulus occurs, organized packets of instruction are supplied from their storage areas in the brain. Teetering on a boulder requires a different set of instructions than stepping on a sharp thorn. The responses to our environment are preset programs of muscular tension fed forward to appropriate body parts. In other words, to continually respond to our changing environment, we need to receive feedback from our senses and to respond with "feed forward" from our brain.

Endorphin Release

The response of the body to pain is an attempt to inhibit it through the release of endorphins, the body's natural pain relievers. The demand of pressure has been linked to endorphin release. Strong tactile stimulation, such as pressure, diminishes pain through competition. The pressure signal competes with the pain signal by blocking the "gate" to the higher levels of the nervous system. Rubbing the feet so dominates the nerve cells affected by pain that the pain messages are inhibited.

Archetype / Archestructure

Archetypes are "symbolic image(s) ... without known origin and they reproduce themselves in any time or in another part of the world – even when transmission by direct descent or 'cross fertilization' through migration must be ruled out." (Carl G. Jung, *Man and His Symbols*, Dell Publishing Co., 1968, p. 58)

"An archestructure can now be defined as a felt or perceived function or structural feature of the nervous system, projected or unconsciously acted out in the life-style or the beliefs, customs and social structures of the individuals concerned or of whole communities." (Stan F. Gooch, *Total Man*, Ballantine Books, 1972, p. 299)

The practice of foot work in a variety of cultures, belief systems, and historical periods speaks of a universal bridging concept. It speaks of an archestructural, physiological need that work on feet helps to fill. The physiological demands of walking upright in a field of gravity creates stress on the body. Such demands link the various attempts throughout history to care for the body through technique applied to the feet.

Throughout history various cultures have utilized the feet as a means of effecting the body and its health. The concept of "working on feet" shows signs of being an archetypical practice. Although varying in detail, it seems to reappear rather than cross-link from another culture. From the Physician's

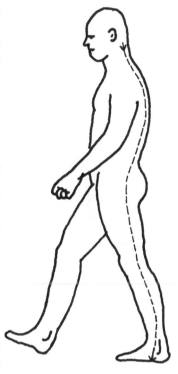

Feed forward: Instructions about the next foot step are relayed from the brain to the foot as well as all other parts of the body.

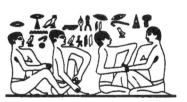

7

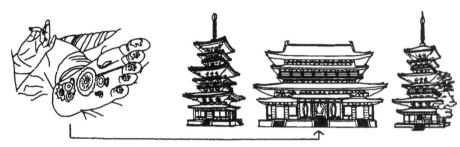

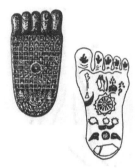

Tomb of ancient Egypt (2300 B. C.) to the Medicine Teacher Temple of Japan (690 A. D.), ancient cultures around the world have practiced some form of foot work. Examples can be found historically in Tibet, India, and China as well.

The current practice of reflexology is a method of utilizing pressure techniques applied to the feet to provoke a response from the entire body. It has its origins in the exploration of the workings of the nervous system and subsequent discovery of the reflex by the medical community in the last half of the 1800's. (See "Influence on the Body Through the Reflexes," p. 11.)

Reflex Stress

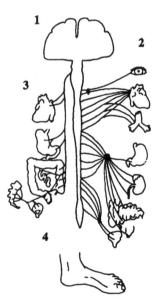

The walking mechanism is inextricably linked to the internal organs. At the same time a sensory organ such as the foot is being sent instructions from the brain, the internal organs are also receiving instructions. These instructions are about the fuel and oxygen necessary to make movement possible. The entire process takes place as an automatic, unconscious response or a reflexive action.

In case of danger, the feet participate in the overall body reaction to ensure the survival of the being. This reaction is commonly known as "fight or flight" because the body gears its internal structures to provide the fuel necessary for either eventuality. Muscles ready for action are also a part of this overall body response. The sudden adrenal surge which enables a person to lift a car is an example of this reaction. In case of danger, the hands reach for a weapon and the feet prepare to fight or flee. Pressure sensors in the feet are a part of the body's reflexive network that makes possible the "fight or flight" response.

Fight or flight response: In case of danger the brain (1) communicates with the internal organs through the autonomic nervous system (2), (3) and the muscles, such as those of the foot through the central nervous system. (4) (See pp. 162-170.)

Just as the foot maintains a level of readiness to meet the demands made on it, the body as a whole stands prepared for any eventuality. Reflex stress is the tension level necessary to achieve the communication between all body parts for highly organized tasks. Preset instructions are "mapped" in the nervous system to direct instant response to any new challenge.

Reflex Area Map

Reflexes are organized responses to stimulus. Stimulus to the surface of the body requires an immediate response to avoid potentially dangerous situations. A poke in the eye is different from a pat on the back. The ability to make such a distinction and to respond appropriately is created by well-rehearsed reflexive responses of the nervous system.

An image of the body is mapped on the brain. This provides a site for analysis of the exact nature and surface location of a stimulus. Sensory information is thus guided to a map in the brain where evaluation of specific information takes place. Sensory stimulation applied to the feet is routed to an area different from that of sensory stimulation applied to the arm. Pressure information from the foot is guided to a part of the brain specializing in interpreting pressure. Stretch, movement, and touch sensations perceived by the foot are routed to neighboring yet separate areas of the brain for analysis.

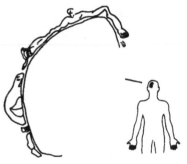

Mapping: Images of the body are mapped on the cortex of the brain to receive information about bodily sensation (sensory cortex) and to provide instructions about muscular activity (motor cortex).

The importance of such mapping is quite simply to keep track of all incoming messages so that any stimulus is connected to the appropriate response. When the proper connection is made, the proper response is made automatically and unconsciously to the particular demand.

As we have said before, every day is not a new day for a sensory organ such as a foot. Just as a filing cabinet holds papers that are needed for future reference, the brain files the information it needs for intended activities such as walking. Fine touch impressions, surface location, body image, and body position are all constructed from information garnered from these "filing cabinets" in the brain. Today's body image is built from yesterday's image and those gathered over a lifetime.

The accumulation of a lifetime of stress and adaptation to stress are reflected in this mapping of the body image. All these reflections, the benefit of past experience, are shared with all body parts to make possible the complex responses to demands. The capability to respond to demands is encoded in these maps as well. Because of the almost instantaneous response needed to meet a demand such as a change in surface underfoot, an established, preset response is on file not only in the brain but also in other body parts that need to know what to do immediately.

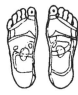

The foot plays a crucial role in the basic survival mechanism of locomotion. An image of the body is mapped on the foot as a game plan of what to do. It is this template of information that makes possible an integrated response to stress. These preset programs ("feed forward" instructions from the brain) maintain a stress level in the foot. The necessary response to an emergency or a day-to-day demand are thus made.

The reflex image on the foot shows a map of adaptation to stress. The map is updated with information continually. The map represents the range within which response or reflexive action can take place. A customized, detailed response to stress reflects the capabilities of the individual. The whole body, feet included, thus receives plans from the brain detailing possible responses. The body is thus prepared to act reflexively through its sensory, locomotive, and autonomic systems to ensure that life goes on.

Mapping: An image of the body is mapped on the foot to reflect a continually updated picture of the body's ability to respond to stress.

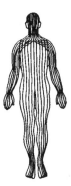

Zonal Maps

Zones recognize the relationship between the demands of gravity and the upright body. Zones are reflected onto the body as a part of the information fed forward from the brain to provide instruction and direction about moving in a field of gravity. Such an organizational scheme on the body mirrors the longitudinal filing system of sensory information in the brain.

Body Stress

"Homeostasis is the state of equilibrium of the internal environment of the body that is maintained by the dynamic processes of feedback and regulation." (*Taber's Cyclopedic Medical Dictionary*, Philadelphia, F. A. Davis, 1981, p. 667)

Body stress is the overall state of equilibrium needed to maintain homeostasis. It is this dynamic state of tension that links us to integrated movement and behavior. It allows us to act as a whole for the goal of purposeful activity. While a state of stress is necessary for life itself, stress without interruption causes wear and tear throughout the body.

Reflexology works because it taps into this basic body stress mechanism. Through the organized application of techniques to the feet, the reflexologist interrupts the pattern of stress created by walking and influences the homeostasis of the body.

10

Influence on the Body Through the Reflexes

Reflexology systems have been created throughout history to impact the dynamic equilibrium of the body. British physicians of the late 1800's created techniques to influence the body through the (then) recently discovered reflex and its reflexive action. Heat, cold, plasters, and herbal poultices were applied to one part of the body to influence another. Such work was considered a cutaneal / visceral response as techniques applied to the skin (cutaneous) produced an effect on an internal body part (viscera).

Russian physicians of the early 1900's followed the reflex research of Nobel Prize winner Ivan Pavlov to create reflex therapy. Their basic idea, to influence reflexes and thus brain-organ dynamics, survives as a medical practice today. To physician-researchers, such as Vladimir Bekterev who coined the word "reflexology" in 1917, an organ experiences illness because it receives the wrong operating instructions from the brain. By interrupting the body's misguided instructions, the reflex therapist prompts the body to behave in a better manner. Conditioning of better behavior is achieved by the application of a series of such interruptions. A stomach ulcer, for example, is treated by applying a series of subcutaneous injections to the abdomen. (An 80% effectiveness rate is reported with best results for those with an ulcer of less than five years duration.)

The introduction of Zone Therapy by Dr. William Fitzgerald, an American physician, in the early 1900's is considered to be influenced by the (then) current studies in Europe into the reflexes. He observed that direct pressure to the body could produce an anesthesia effect. His further findings that direct pressure also caused a therapeutic effect created controversy in the medical community. His Zone Therapy model was not universally accepted. While flourishing for a period of time among a portion of the med-

BRAIN.

JULY, 1878.

Original Articles.

REFLEX ACTION AS A CAUSE OF DISEASE AND MEANS OF CURE.

BY T. LAUDER BRUNTON, M.D., F.R.S.[1]

A

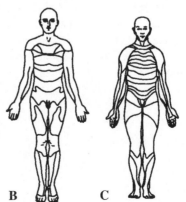

B   C

Reflexive Influences: Reflexive action as a method of influencing the body has been explored throughout history including nineteenth century:
A British neurological researchers of 1878
B Head's Zones of 1893
C dermatomes of 1919

Zonal Influences

Various therapeutic uses of zones to influence the body were developed in the early 1900's, such as:

D Fitzgerald's Zones of 1914
E Riley's zones extended into the foot and

F Hirata's Zones from Japan of 1911.

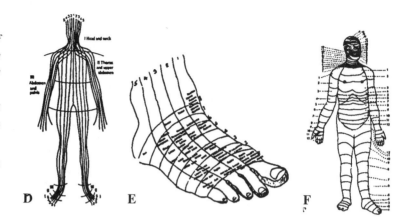

D   E   F

ical community, his ideas were eliminated with other "drugless" modalities of treatment when drugs and surgical procedures became the primary means of treatment. His ideas were carried on through the work of individuals such as Dr. Joseph Riley and physio-therapist Eunice Ingham who applied Zone Therapy to the feet. Ingham's original model included recognition of a reflexive response within the nervous system of the body to application of pressure to the feet. She later abandoned this explanation in response to legal pressures of the times. She is recognized, however, for developing and keeping alive the ideas of zone therapy and reflexology in the United States.

Kunz and Kunz theorized independently (Paralysis Report, 1981) that reflexology techniques influence the body through the autonomic / somatic integration that takes place when the internal organs adjust to sensory input. In work with three paralyzed individuals over a three-year period, we found that the application of pressure techniques to particular parts of the foot elicited particular movement of the opposing foot or hand. Over time the random spastic movement became sophisticated movement recognizable as a portion of the stride mechanism. Also, the general response to pressure technique application was a stereotypical response of the body's basic regulating mechanism, the autonomic nervous system. One individual shivered and experienced chattering teeth. Another perspired on one side of his head. The third experienced gastro-intestinal grumbling as well as perspiration below the level of the spinal cord injury.

A Stress Model of the Body

To explain the impact of reflexes and reflexive actions on the homeostasis of the body, Hans Selye, noted stress researcher, proposed a theory of general adaptation to stress. In the 1920's he noted that burn patients frequently suffered from stomach ulcers. The burns, thus, had an effect on the body quite distant from the site of the injury. From further studies, Selye came to view the burns and other demands on the body as stressors. He found that the body reacts to stress in a predictable manner. He called this predictable reaction a General Adaptation to Stress.

Selye describes stress as a three-stage process. Whether it is the life-threatening stress of falling into an icy lake or the stress of day-to-day life, stress over time follows a pattern of initial alarm, subsequent adaptation, and eventual exhaustion. During the alarm stage, the body is seen as adjusting to a new stressor. During the adaptation phase, the stressor has been present for a sufficient enough time to become ingrained in the brain-organ dynamics, altering the function of the body. During the exhaustion phase, the response to stress has been conditioned over an extended period of time. It results in an alteration of both function and structure of the body.

If the body is subjected to regular doses of stress over time, the effects are cumulative and it becomes more and more difficult to return to homeostasis. Here, some researchers estimate, is the root cause of 80% of all illness. Selye found that it is not stress itself but the continuous nature of the stress that creates wear and tear on the body. He links prolonged stress to stress-related illnesses. In addition, he discovered that the body has only so much "adaptive energy" with which to respond to stress. Once this finite amount of energy is used, exhaustion results.

General Adaptive Syndrome (Selye)

Adaptive Stage	Characteristics	Age of Life
Alarm	"The body shows the changes characteristic of the first exposure to a stressor."	Childhood
Resistance	"Resistance ensues if continued exposure to the stressor is compatible with adaptation."	Adulthood
Exhaustion	"Following long-continued exposure to the same stressor, to which the body has become adjusted, eventually adaptive energy is exhausted."	Old Age

From Hans Selye's *Stress Without Distress*, New York, New American Library, 1974, p. 27

Interruption of Stress Through Reflexology

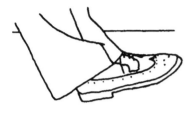

Shoes and flat surfaces add to the stress of walking. The foot over-uses certain of its locomotive capabilities and under-uses others. Inefficiency in the stride mechanism drains from the finite energy available to each of us for stress adaptation and lessens the energy available for other functions.

Reflexology techniques provide a variety of sensory experiences and demands which interrupt the patterns of stress created by walking. The applications of technique are requests in the body's own language of proprioception. The foot is used as a keyboard to ask the body to interrupt its present stress programming and pay attention to the demands of pressure technique application. The adaptation to this stimulus is a form of learning. As in any learning situation, the consistency and frequency of technique application play a role in the learning process.

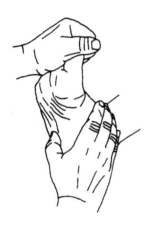

Through practice of the foot's full capabilities, stress is interrupted. With consistent technique application over time, the body is conditioned to make the best possible adaptation to stress. Ongoing technique application creates an educational experience.

Reflexology technique application interrupts the cycle of stress by creating a set of demands on the body apart from the mundane, everyday experiences. The goal of the reflexologist is to apply pressure techniques for the purpose of interrupting stress and provoking response within the dynamics of the stress mechanism. In addition, with technique applied over time, the stress mechanism is conditioned to behave in a manner that creates less wear and tear on the body.

Applied Theory

Reflexology is the organized, systematic application of pressure technique to the feet. Technique is applied on the basis of evaluation of the individual's feet, which reflect a body image formed by adaptation to stress. The foot reflects the body's response to the stresses of gravity and movement. Technique is applied according to two body images of stress adaptation: zones and areas. Zones are a recognition that all body parts must move in relationship to gravity. Reflex areas recognize that to move, all body parts must act in relationship to each other. The reflexology and zone charts thus denote the dynamics of the body's stress mechanism, one part responding to gravity and the other to movement. The feet reflect in an organized manner the stress mechanism and thus the overall level of stress.

Think of a slide or a movie projector. The projector projects a picture onto a screen. And you can make adjustments if the picture is blurry. The brain serves as a projector. It projects instructions down the spinal cord and throughout the nervous system about how the body is to operate. It is, in essence, projecting an image of how the body should work. Each body part receives instructions appropriate to its task. The kidneys, for example, are sent directions about their job of elimination of waste products and mineral balance. The feet receive information about locomotion as well as information about the whole body, so that their activities can match the abilities of other body parts to fight or flee. It is these shared images or projections of instructions from the brain that make integrated activities possible.

Reflex images or maps are projected throughout the body to routinely coordinate the activities of the body. An image of longitudinal zones is projected from the brain to the body to provide instructions about an upright alignment in response to gravity. An image of the body is projected onto the feet to provide instantaneous, detailed directions about responding to the demands of walking, running, or any of the other facets of the basic survival mechanism of locomotion.

Zone Theory

Zone theory is the basis of foot reflexology. Reflexology has become a more refined system, but zone theory is still a useful adjunct to it. An understanding of it is essential to an understanding of reflexology. Zones are a system for organizing relationships between various parts of the body. They can be thought of as guidelines, or markers, which link one part to another.

There are ten equal longitudinal zones running the length of the body from the top of the head to the tips of the toes. (See Illus.) The number ten corresponds to the number of fingers and toes and therefore provides a convenient numbering system. Each finger and each toe falls into one zone, with the left thumb, for example, occurring in the same zone as the left big toe, and so on.

Using the zone chart, trace the ten zones on your own body. Begin with your feet and trace imaginary lines from each toe up the leg, through the trunk of the body, to the top of the head. Each toe represents a zone. Do the same exercise with the hands. Begin tracing from each finger. Note on the

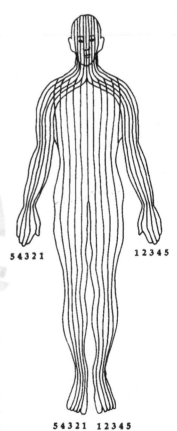

54321   12345

54321 12345

chart how the numbered zones intersect with each other in the neck and head area.

Each big toe corresponds to half of the head area, even though it also represents one specific zone as well. But each big toe also represents the four smaller toes, in that the little toes occupy the remaining zones which represent the head/neck region in finer terms. This concept is fully explained in Reflexology Theory.

Like an arrow passing through, the reflex points are considered to pass all the way through the body within the same zones. The same point, for instance, can be found on the front as well as on the back of the body, on the top as well as on the bottom of the foot.

Adaptation to stress in any part of a zone will affect the entire zone running through the whole length of the body. Sensitivity in a specific part of the foot signals the reflexologist that there is something going on in that zone or zones somewhere in the body. Direct pressure applied to any part of a zone will affect the entire zone. This is the basis of zone theory. It is also the basis of foot reflexology, because not only are the feet functional parts of the body with representation in each of the zones, they are a direct reiteration of the body itself. They actually mirror the body (see p. 16). However, working the entire foot affects the entire body. Because of the myriad of zonal relationships, it is always valuable to work the entire foot.

There are other reasons that the feet are able to serve in this capacity. They are a very sensitive part of the zonal system. Besides being "sheltered" constantly by shoes and socks, this terminal end of the body plays a particularly important role in gathering pressure information necessary for walking.

Reflex Areas

In addition to the longitudinal zones of zone theory, reflexology also uses the lateral zones on the body. Their main purpose is to help fix the image of the body onto the feet in the proper perspective and location. Only three lateral zones are commonly used: shoulder line, diaphragm line, and waistline. However, the concept of lateral zones applies to all areas.

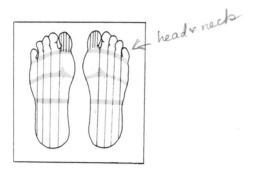

head & neck

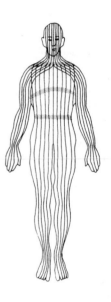

For example, consider the portion of the body above the shoulders, the head and neck region. Zone theory tells us that all ten zones of the body run through this region. As we have pointed out, each big toe represents half of the head, with the dual role of occupying zone one and at the same time representing all five zones. (See Illus.) The small toes on each foot are a zonal breakdown of their respective big toe. As such, they define the head / neck region in finer terms. (The ball of each small toe represents part of the head, whereas the stem corresponds to part of the neck.) This allows us to visualize the physical image of the body on the feet. Relationships and juxtapositions of body parts can be traced on the feet as they occur in the body itself.

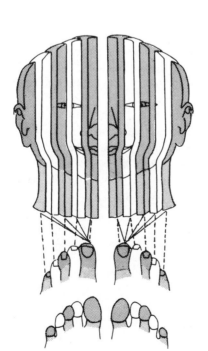

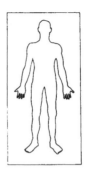

The above illustration is a two-dimensional representation of the body. Even though it is flat, we interpret the image as a three-dimensional one. Any chart representing the reflexes on the feet should be interpreted in the same way. Therefore, the parts of the body "projected" onto the feet (see chart) are considered to be three-dimensional too. Since the feet are not flat (obvious, but we couldn't resist the pun), projecting onto the feet means there is depth to the picture. We are merely dealing with the *surface* of the feet. The reflexes actually pass through the areas where they are depicted. To help you visualize the image of the body on the feet, try this exercise: Ask a friend to volunteer a pair of feet. First, look at the bottoms of the two feet placed side by side so that they are touching. Imagine you are looking at the trunk of a body from the front. You can't see the spine from in front but you know it's there, dividing the body in half. The spine would occur "between" the two feet to be consistent with our image, But each foot represents one half of the body (right foot = right side, left foot = left side), so the spine itself is divided in half with each foot having a spinal area along the inside edge.

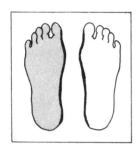

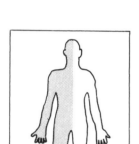

The head is the top of the body. On your trunk, visualize it where the big toes are. Each big toe represents half of the head and neck. The ball of the toe is the head itself and the stem is the neck. Think of each as a slice of the head and neck. The ridge at the base of the toes corresponds to the top of the trunk, the shoulder line. The shoulder joints occur on the outside, below the little toe in the ball of each foot.

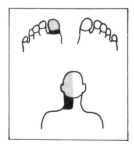

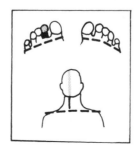

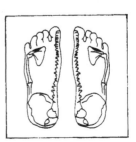

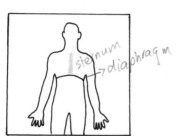

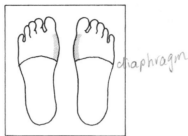

To locate the solar plexus area on the feet, first find the sternum on your own body. This is the bone in the middle of your chest connecting the two rib cages. At the base of the sternum is where the diaphragm is attached. Now add it to your picture of the trunk on the two feet. Your diaphragm line should have included the area extending all the way across the base of the ball of each foot.

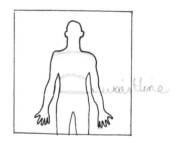

On the outside of the foot, about halfway down, is a protruding bone called the fifth metatarsal. If you were to draw a line all the way around the foot at this bone, you would have a good image of the waistline. Below this line are such parts of the anatomy as the lower back, hips, and intestines. On the feet, the reflexes corresponding to these as well as all other parts of the anatomy below the waist are located below this line.

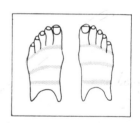

Next look at the tops of your own feet as they rest together. Visualize the back view of the trunk of a body projected onto them. The spine, of course, runs down the inside of each foot. The back of the head is represented by the two big toes. And the shoulder line runs along the base of the toes. Now extend the diaphragm line around from the bottoms of each foot across the tops. Do the same with the waistline, at the fifth metatarsal. These represent important boundaries and will help you properly locate the rest of the anatomy within these guidelines. For example, the area of the back between the bottom of the shoulder blades and the top of the shoulder is bounded by the diaphragm line on the bottom and the shoulder line on top. Any parts of the anatomy occurring in this area of the trunk will have reflexes on the feet between these two lines.

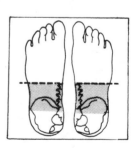

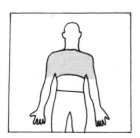

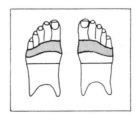

19

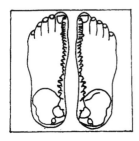

The pelvis is attached at the spine and curves around to create an area with depth (as you can see on your own body). Similarly on the feet, the area representing the hip / pelvis can be seen as three-dimensional. This area curves around the foot, covering the base of the ankle, around the ankle bones themselves, and the sides and bottoms of the foot.

Although the model we have just described is useful for conceiving the locations of the major lateral zones, do NOT think of the bottom of the foot ONLY as the front of the body or the top of the foot ONLY as the back of the body. Both the top and bottom of the foot represent the front and back of the body as well as the organs in between. In other words, the reflexes pass through the feet.

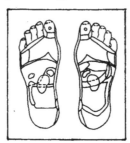 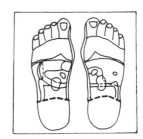

The Internal Organs

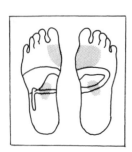

If you have seen standard anatomy charts in any encyclopedia or textbook, you may have noticed that internal organs lay on top of, lap over, behind, between, and against each other in every possible configuration. The areas on the feet corresponding to them must then overlap as well. This is quite difficult to represent accurately on a foot chart. The heart, for instance, is more or less to the left of the midline of the body, but it extends into the right side also. There must be a small area then, on the right foot corresponding to this portion.

It is important to maintain the image on the foot of a three-dimensional representation of a three-dimensional body. The kidney area on the chart overlaps with many other areas just as the kidneys overlap other organs and parts of the body when viewed from back or front. Remember that the chart is designed for convenience and clarity. Once you have a solid picture of the body projected onto the feet, you will know that you are actually working through multiple reflex areas throughout much of the trunk area of the body.

Foot Reflexology Chart

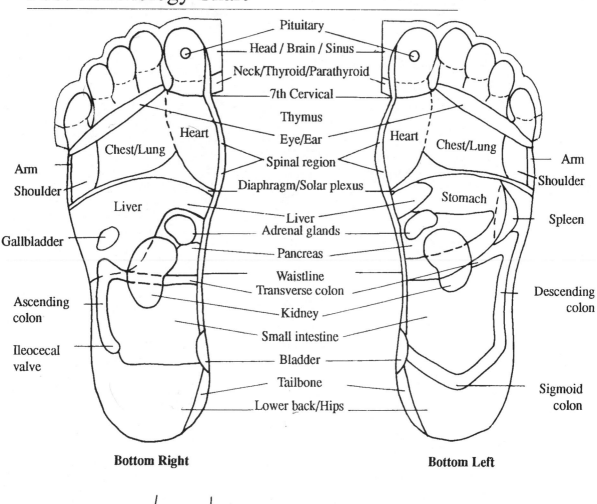

Bottom Right

Bottom Left

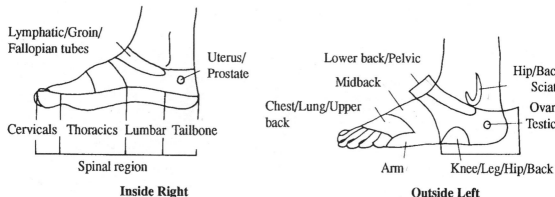

Inside Right

Outside Left

21

Foot Reflexology Chart

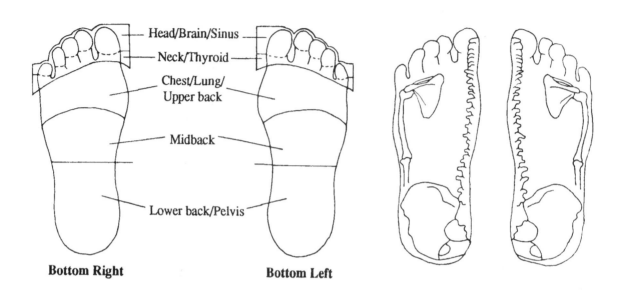

Bottom Right   **Bottom Left**

Head/Brain/Sinus
Neck/Thyroid
Chest/Lung/Upper back
Midback
Lower back/Pelvis

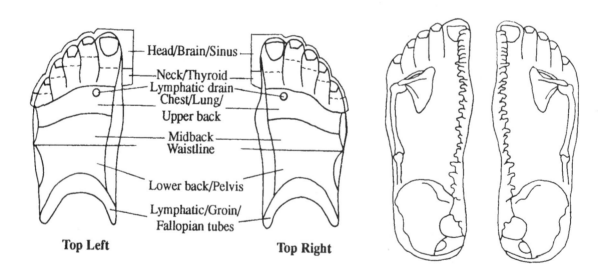

Top Left   **Top Right**

Head/Brain/Sinus
Neck/Thyroid
Lymphatic drain
Chest/Lung/Upper back
Midback
Waistline
Lower back/Pelvis
Lymphatic/Groin/Fallopian tubes

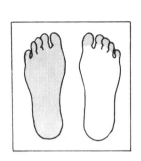 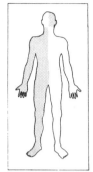 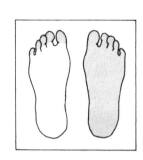 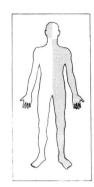

Important Exception to the Zonal Concept

The most fundamental zonal concept is that the right foot represents the right side of the body, and the left foot the left side. There is an important exception, however. In the central nervous system, the right half of the brain controls the left side of the body and vice versa. So in any disorders or problems affecting the brain or central nervous system (i.e., stroke, paralysis, etc.), emphasize the appropriate area of the foot on the opposite side from the trauma or injury.

Guidelines

The midline refers to the line dividing the body in half from top to bottom. It is represented by the separation of the feet. Approaching the midline describes movement toward the inside of the foot (arch). Working away from the midline denotes movement toward the outside of the foot.

Uses of Zone Theory in Reflexology

It is a common assumption that the hands and feet are the only areas to which the techniques of reflexology can be applied effectively. Actually, there are reflexes throughout the zones of the body. It is important to understand the zonal system because it will explain the unlikely relationships within zones. It is a valuable enhancement to the regular repertoire of techniques and applications.

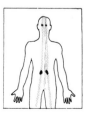

An excellent example of the unusual relationships that are revealed with the zonal system is the relationship between the eyes and the kidneys. Because they both lie in the same zones, working the kidney areas of the feet has been helpful in many cases of eye disorder.

23

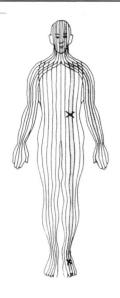

Practical uses of zone theory include using the zones to find an area on the foot representing a pain or injury elsewhere in the body and using a system we call "referral areas." Sometimes when a medical diagnosis has not been possible, a *generalized* pain somewhere in the body can be traced using the zones to a *distinct* area on the foot. It can then be worked by emphasizing that particular area of the foot.

As a practice exercise, look at the illustration. Notice the spot marked "x" where, let's say, there's some pain or injury. By tracing along the appropriate zone down into the foot, you can find sensitivity there too. Since the basic principle of reflexology is that buildup will occur in that zone of the foot as a result of the stress or injury in spot "x," the zonal relationships provide guidelines for locating more pain more precisely. Using this information source in conjunction with the lateral zones on the feet permits the reflexologist to concentrate the effort on special target areas to relieve the trauma.

Referral Areas

An injury on the foot should never be worked on. This includes varicose veins, phlebitis, sprained ankle, or any limb or joint injury. Reflexology and zone theory allow us to select alternate parts of the body in the same zones and work them instead. This system is called "referral areas." Referral areas are different parts of the body that relate to each other through the zones. They are very valuable because of what they tell us about what is going on in the zones. They also provide excellent areas for self-help homework, so that the client can amplify the reflexologist's efforts between treatments. When an area must be avoided entirely (due to an injury), the referral area is the alternative for working the zone.

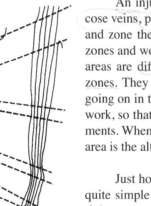

Referral Areas
shoulder......hip
upper arm ......thigh
elbow......knee
forearm......calf
wrist......ankle
hand......foot
fingers......toes

Just how the limbs are related to each other through the zones is really quite simple. Each relationship is specialized. For example, compare your right arm and leg to the illustration. The arm is a reflection of the leg in zone terms. The fingers correspond to the toes, the hand to the foot, the wrist to the ankle, the forearm to the calf, the elbow to the knee, the upper arm to the thigh and the shoulder to the hip. If any part of the arm is injured, the corresponding part of the leg can be worked (and vice versa). Common problems such as phlebitis and varicose veins in the legs can be helped by working the same general areas of the arms.

Practice using the referral areas. To begin, set up the zones to get your bearings. Place your hands palms down on your knees. Number the zones starting with the thumb and big toe (Zone 1), the index finger and second toe (Zone 2), and so forth. Your picture may get a little distorted, though, because the arm and leg bend in "different" directions. When you placed your hands palms down, you rotated the radius bone of the arm. Now turn your hands over, palms up, and notice that the arm is straight but the zones no longer match. The thumb now seems to be in the same zone as the *little* toe. But it isn't. Use this perspective only to help you accurately find the part of the referral area to work.

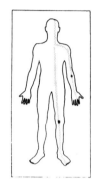

Look at the illustration. Where would you work for an injury to the inside of the left knee? Which zone is it in? Since it is in line with the second toe, we will call it "Zone 2." Hold your left hand palm up. Start with the second finger and trace Zone 2 up to the elbow. This would be your referral area for this particular knee injury. If you actually did encounter an injury here, you would probably find tenderness in the referral area of the elbow.

The same approach can be used to locate other referral areas. Identify which zone(s) an injury has occurred in and simply trace it to the referral area. Often the tenderness in the referral area will help you find it. With your hand palm up you can see that, contradictory as it may seem, the fleshy part of the forearm is the referral area for the fleshy part of the calf of the leg. The bony part of the forearm corresponds to the shin. The same holds true for the upper arm and thigh, with the front of the thigh corresponding to the triceps (back) of the arm.

The importance of referral areas cannot be exaggerated. They can give insights into the problem areas by showing the relationships to the areas in the same zone(s) that may be at the root of a problem. Take a shoulder problem, for example. Because the shoulder lies in the same zone as the hip, a hip problem could be aggravating the shoulder. Referral areas point out just one more way the body operates as a whole.

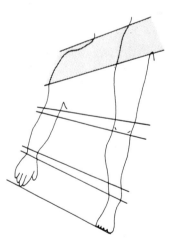

The finger and thumb walking techniques can be adapted for use in working referral areas on the body. Often it is most efficient to walk all four fingers side by side through an area. When working a referral area on the knee or elbow, remember that the reflexes do pass through. Instead of trying to work the bony side (kneecap or elbow bone), find the corresponding area in the soft, fleshy crook of the joint.

In Summary

The body acts as an integrated whole in response to stress. All body systems act together to maintain the body's natural equilibrium, its homeostasis. The feet play a significant role in this communication system. The role of the feet is to act reflexively, automatically, and unconsciously to particular demands. The physiological demands of walking upright in a field of gravity link the application of reflexology technique to its influence on the body, the interruption of stress. A structural system exists in the nervous system to manage these activities. The goals of reflexology are to condition and exercise the nervous system so that it will respond in a better manner to the demands of the day.

In this book, you will acquire the skills to influence health through reflexology. Our goal is to provide you with the information you need as the complete reflexologist: the skillful practitioner, successful business person and respected professional. The skills you will acquire provide the basis for the services you will furnish to your clientele. The goals of services are multi-fold: relaxation, body awareness, assessment, exercise of pressure sensors, and targeting stress-related health concerns.

To provide such services, you will learn how to apply the appropriate amount of the right technique to the proper reflex areas to create the changes sought by the client. In addition, you will learn how to provide a reflexology assessment, that unique picture of what's going on with the client's stress pattern. You will see that it is your ability to communicate your work that will be of value to your client, other professionals and those who pay for expert services such as insurers. Such skills are complemented by knowledge of theory, history, research, professionalism, business, anatomy, physiology, and reflex areas related to disorders.

With such skills, you can become a successful professional and expert in a unique and valued field. As continuing research reveals the full potential of reflexology work, reflexologists will increasingly provide a complement to medical care, furnishing a unique, safe, and effective path to health.

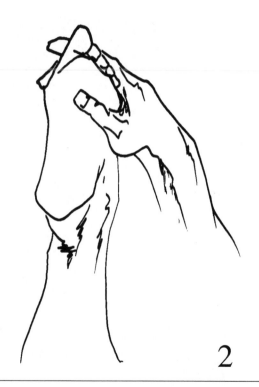

2

Techniques

Techniques

The techniques described in this chapter are designed to achieve two main goals: efficiency and effectiveness in applying pressure technique to the feet. In reflexology, efficiency is covering a reflex area with the least amount of effort. Effectiveness is hitting the points, being dead-on-target in every reflex area.

Getting Started

Before you begin your practice of techniques, you will want to prepare yourself and your work area. Both you and the person with whom you work should be comfortable. First, wash your hands thoroughly. Since fingernails should never make contact with the foot, you'll want to trim yours to be no longer than the tips of the fingers. An optimal working position for you will be one where your hands rest on the individual's feet with your elbows bent at a 90° angle. Seating on a lower chair will help or the feet can be raised by resting them on a pillow. Seating in a recliner will be comfortable for the individual. If not available, use seating where the individual's knees and back are supported.

Basic Techniques

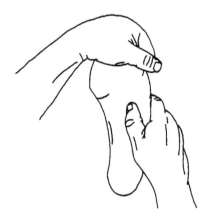

The three basic techniques are the *thumb walking,* the *finger walking,* and the *thumb hook and back up*. Proper thumb motion covers large areas efficiently. *Finger walking* is a fine-tuning technique for the tops and sides of the feet. The *hook and back up* pinpoints specific, hard to reach reflex areas.

The three motions combined with leverage and proper holding of the foot form the basis of the techniques used in foot reflexology. One hand is a "working" hand while the other is a "holding" hand. The working hand does the *thumb* and *finger walking* and *the hook and back up* techniques. Each of the techniques has its own special holding problems. Detailed information on holding techniques is given with each technique section. In general, a stationary target is easier to hit than a moving one. So in reflexology, a stationary foot can be more effectively worked. You must, then, become aware of how your holding hand is contributing to your effectiveness.

Holding the Foot

Holding the foot properly contributes to the overall effectiveness and efficiency of the three basic techniques. Proper holding facilitates walking with the thumb or fingers because it provides a stationary target and thins out the flesh so that the reflex points can be reached. The hand responsible for holding the foot in all of the techniques will hereafter be called the "holding" hand.

The Thumb Walking Technique

The *thumb walking* technique has a very simple basis: the bending of the first joint of the thumb. Try this exercise: hold the thumb below the first joint (as shown). This prevents the second joint from bending. Bend the first joint. Do it several times. Now try the other thumb.

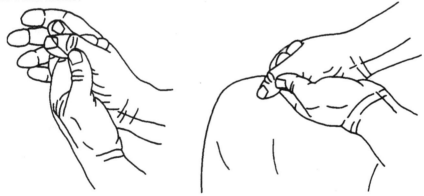

While you're still holding, place the outside corner of the thumb on your leg. Bend the thumb a few times. At this point, do not worry about exerting pressure or about what your other fingers are doing.

The next step is to get the thumb actually walking forward. Hold on to your thumb. Use the outside tip. Bend the thumb, allowing it to rock a little from the thumb tip to the lower edge of the thumb nail. This is not a large range of motion: it is not meant to be.

Remove the holding hand. Try walking the thumb. Are you bending only the first joint? Do not push the thumb forward. Bending and unbending is the entire means by which you move forward.

It is at this point in our discussion of technique that an important aspect of efficiency arises. The fact is that actual strength in reflexology comes from the use of LEVERAGE. In the *thumb walking* technique, leverage is attained by the use of the four fingers in opposition to the thumb.

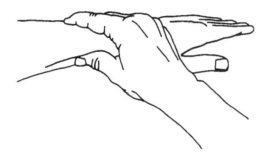 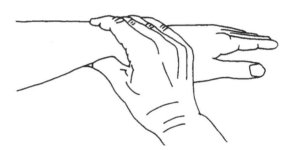

To practice using leverage, place the four fingers of the working hand on the opposite forearm (as shown). Keep the fingers and hand in the position shown. Lower the wrist of the working hand. You will be pulling and holding on with the four fingers while the thumb is pressed into the forearm. Maintain this position with the wrist lowered and allow the thumb to walk. Note the increased pressure now exerted by the thumb. The leverage provided by the fingers and the position of the wrist regulate the strength of the thumb. So the rule of leverage for thumb walking is: **Raise the wrist, lower the pressure. Lower the wrist, increase the pressure.**

Refining the Thumb Walking Technique

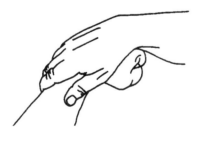

It is essential to walk the thumb with a constant, steady pressure. Practice on your forearm. Walk the thumb, taking smaller and smaller "bites." Practice until you feel the steady pressure. **You should not feel an on-off-on-off pressure at each bend of the thumb.**

Finally, achieving good leverage means learning the proper *angle* of the thumb. Lay your hands down on a table or flat surface. Note how the thumb rests on the table. Walk it in this relaxed position. The outside edge now making contact with the table is the part of the thumb that should make contact with the foot. It can be described as the area from the lower outside edge of the nail to the tip of the thumb. By using this portion of the thumb correctly, you take best advantage of the leverage available from the four fingers.

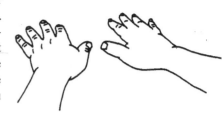

Applying Thumb Walking to the Feet

Now let's apply to the feet what we have learned. The thumb walking technique is most effective for covering the large reflex areas on the bottom of the feet. There is quite a bit of flesh between your thumb and the reflex points. Therefore, the holding hand will be used for foot control, to thin the flesh out, and to give the thumb a chance to work the necessary reflex areas. In most instances this means holding the toes back with the holding hand.

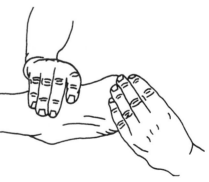

With the holding hand, grasp the toes of a friend's foot. Hold them back (as shown). Feel for the tendon with your working hand. Avoid it for the moment. Now practice walking with the thumb on the bottom of the foot. Are you applying a constant, steady pressure? Remember: The thumb ALWAYS moves forward, NEVER backwards or sideways.

While your thumb is walking on the bottom of the foot, notice what your leverage fingers are doing. They should be in a firm but natural position. If the thumb begins to walk away from this natural hand position, the hand is stretched out and leverage is lost. It is necessary to constantly reposition the fingers to maintain the essential leverage. Incidentally, the four fingers work as a unit and should be kept together. When the fingers are spread apart, some effectiveness is lost. If one or more fingers is lifted off the surface, even more leverage effectiveness is lost.

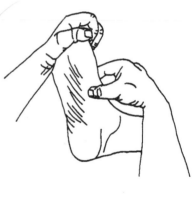

Note the angle of your moving thumb in relationship to the surface of the foot. The thumb moves within a small range of motion, from a position of a 10° angle to a 20° angle as it walks. The thumb is always slightly bent to protect it from the strain of over-extension.

31

It will take practice to perfect your technique. Don't be discouraged. This is a whole new thing for your thumb to learn. Be patient and keep trying.

Trouble Shooting/Sore Thumbs/ The Finer Points of Leverage

If you have difficulty with your *thumb walking* technique or if your use of leverage is inadequate, several problems will arise. You may not hit the point effectively. You may rock the thumb too far and hit the foot with the thumb nail. And your thumbs may get sore.

Sore thumbs aren't necessarily a sign of poor technique because building strength in the thumb takes time. But sore thumbs may well point to weaknesses that can easily be corrected by reviewing the technique. Are you trying to press your thumb at each bite? If so, your thumb has every right to be sore! Test your thumb technique on your forearm or on someone else. Are you giving a feeling of on-off-on-off pressure? How much are you bending that first joint? If you're bending to the point that the nail hits the skin, back off a little. (See illus.)

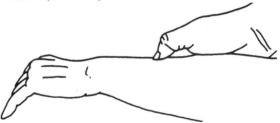

Rethink the thumb technique. Bend your thumb again from the first joint. Practice taking smaller and smaller bites until you can do it with constant, steady pressure. It cannot be over-emphasized. If you don't get it in one or two practice sessions, don't be discouraged. Keep trying. This is the basis for all walking techniques and must be mastered.

When you trouble-shoot your technique, think first of the cardinal rule: **Constant, steady pressure combined with leverage allows you to effectively and efficiently hit the points.** If it seems to you that you *are* exerting this pressure but you still have problems, reevaluate your leverage.

Now let's review the finer points of leverage. First, leverage is what your fingers do to help a walking thumb. When your thumb is walking, the fingers should be contoured to the shape of the foot. This permits you to use the strength of the whole finger. If the fingers are too curled, you use only the strength of each fingertip.

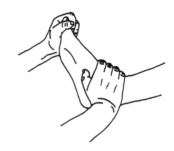

The four fingers should be kept together comfortably. When the fingers are spread out, some leverage is lost. The angle of the thumb also affects your leverage. Once again, using the corner of the thumb allows the most effective opposition to the fingers, thereby utilizing the natural strengths in the hand and fingers.

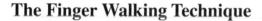

Each of the above considerations adds to the other to produce optimum leverage effectiveness. If you miss any one of the finer points, it detracts a bit from the most effective leverage.

The Finger Walking Technique

The finger walking technique has the same basis as the thumb: the bending of the first joint of the finger. Hold below the first joint (as shown). Bend the first joint.

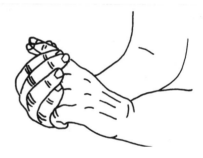

The top of the hand is a good practice ground for finger walking. Try bending from the first joint of the index finger as its tip rests on top of the hand. Use the edge of the finger. The walking motion is a slight rocking from the fingertip to the lower edge of the fingernail.

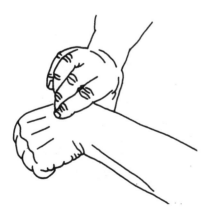

In the *finger walking* technique, good leverage is attained by the use of the thumb in opposition to the fingers. To practice using leverage, place the four fingers of the working hand on the opposite forearm (as shown). Keep the fingers and hand in the position shown. Raise the wrist of the working hand. You should be pulling and holding on with the thumb. The fingers are pressed into the forearm. Maintain this position with the wrist raised, and allow the index finger to walk. Note the increased pressure now exerted by the finger. The leverage provided by the thumb and the position of the wrist regulate the strength of the finger. So the rule of leverage for the *finger walking* technique is: **Raise the wrist, increase the pressure. Lower the wrist, lower the pressure.**

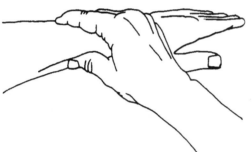
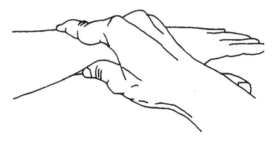

Practice this as you will all techniques. The goal is the same as with the thumb. Take smaller and smaller bites by exerting a constant, steady pressure. Avoid the on-off type of pressure. Remember, the finger always moves in a forward direction, never backwards or sideways.

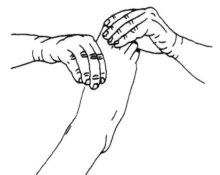

Only one finger at a time does the actual walking. You need not use only the index finger. Any finger can effectively perform the technique.

While one finger is walking, the other fingers contribute to the leverage by following along.

Problems can occur. Usually they involve difficulty in bending the first joint. Try to avoid the following: moving your hand excessively when walking the finger; digging the fingernail into the skin; allowing the walking finger to draw back rather than exerting a constant, forward pressure; merely rolling the walking finger from side to side. If you encounter any of these difficulties, review your technique by closely rereading the description of the technique.

The Hook and Back Up Technique / Pinpointing

The *hook and back up* technique is used to hit a particular point rather than to cover a large reflex area. It is a relatively stationary technique.

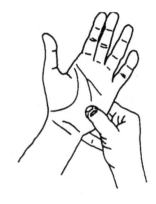

Rest your thumb on the palm of the other hand. Bring your fingers into contact with the top of the hand. Bend the first joint of the thumb, exerting pressure with the corner of the thumb just as you would with the *thumb walking* technique. Now pull back across the point with the thumb. This is the **hook and back up** technique.

As with all techniques, leverage is extremely important in hitting these deeper points. Just as in the case of *thumb walking,* leverage is provided by the fingers and the position of the wrist. (Lower the wrist of the working hand, and the pressure exerted by the thumb is increased. Maintain this position with the wrist lowered. Hook in with the thumb and pull back across the point.

A term that will be used to describe working the deep, specific points of the feet is **pinpointing**. Since no walking is effective on such a small point, the *hook and back up* technique is used.

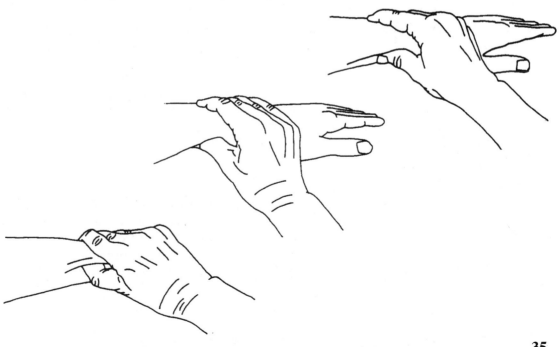

Desserts

Desserts are movement techniques applied by the reflexologist to relax the foot. They bring down the overall tension level. This tension reduction adds greater depth to the reflexology experience. In addition, your job as a reflexologist is made easier as the relaxed foot is more receptive to technique application and you can approach sensitive reflex areas more readily.

Desserts provide a transition between the application of technique to different parts of the foot, and they also serve as instant relaxation for a reflex area sensitive to pressure. The modern-day foot is limited in its stretch and movement by confining shoes and hard surfaces, and desserts create practice and exercise for the stretch and movement sensors in the foot. To assess the application of the dessert, the reflexologist considers how easily the foot moves in the direction encouraged by the dessert.

Side to Side Technique

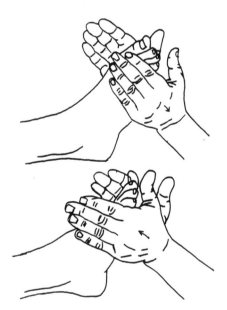

The goal of the side to side technique is to move the foot rhythmically from side to side. The foot is provided exercise of two of its four directions, inversion (inward) and eversion (outward) movements that are normally restricted by flat surfaces and shoe wear. To practice the side to side technique, place your hands on either side of the foot (as shown). The palms of the hands should be in contact with the sides of the foot. Turn the foot from side to side, working the foot back and forth. As the right hand moves one side of the foot away from you, the left hand moves the other side of the foot away from you. Avoid attempting to force the foot to turn farther than is comfortable for the individual. Maintain the position of the hands on the foot. The hands are held in a relaxed yet fixed position. Overly relaxed hands slip on the foot, while rigidly held hands can be abrasive to the foot.

In evaluating the application of the technique, consider whether the foot moves easily from side to side or whether your efforts to move the foot meet with resistance.

Foot Flicking

The goal of foot flicking is to move the foot rapidly and rhythmically in an up-and-down motion. The foot is provided with the exercise of its up (dorsiflexion) and down (plantarflexion) movements. Cup the heel of the foot with the holding hand to provide a base of support as the foot bends at the ankle. The thumb of the working hand is placed on the ball of the foot. The index and middle fingers are placed on top of the foot, opposite the thumb. Your working hand now grasps the head of the first metatarsal bone. With the holding hand, pull slightly on the foot. Push up with the thumb of the working hand and then down with the fingers. Move the foot more and more quickly in a rhythmic movement. Do not force the foot to move. The practice of movement is the goal. In a similar manner, apply the technique to each of the metatarsal heads.

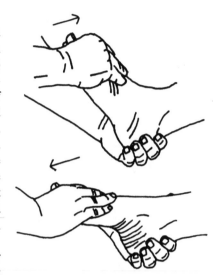

In evaluating the application of the technique, consider whether the foot moves up and down with ease or whether you meet resistance to movement.

Ankle Rotation

This dessert is designed to provide a precise method of rotating the ankles. The goal of technique application is to turn the foot and create a full range of movement for the four major muscle groups connecting foot and leg. Use the left hand to grasp the right foot around the ankle and vice versa. Wrap the fingers around the heel so that the thumb rests in the lymphatic reflex area around the ankle. Grasp with even pressure. With the other hand, grasp the foot below the base of the big toe on the inside of the foot. Once again, use even pressure when holding the foot. Draw a circle in the air with the big toe, rotating the foot in a full 360° circle. Maintain a constant pressure of movement throughout each rotation. Rotate in a clockwise direction and then a counterclockwise direction. Do not grasp the toes.

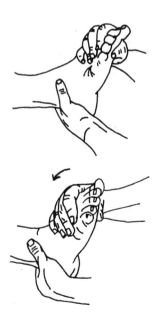

Consider the application of technique as providing an assessment of the lower back and hip reflex areas. In evaluating the application of technique, do you find that the foot moves easily in a full circle or do you meet resistance to movement?

Ankle Traction

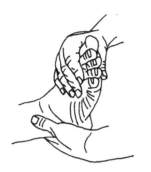

Grasp the foot, cupping the heel with one hand and grasping the ball of the foot. Pull the foot toward you gently and gradually. Hold the foot in a stretched position for ten to fifteen seconds. Hold the technique longer if the individual enjoys the technique.

In evaluating the application of technique, consider the ease with which the foot moves. Does the foot stretch and relax at the ankle or is it tight and constricted?

Toe Rotation

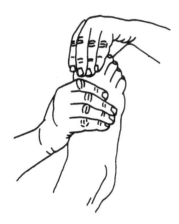

The principles of toe rotation are identical to those of ankle rotation. The goal is the same for the joints of the toes as it is for the ankles during ankle rotation. Place the fingers on the toe (as shown). The fingertips should extend almost to the base of the toe. Using firm, even pressure with the grasping fingers and a slight upward pull, rotate the toe slowly and evenly in full 360° turns. Rotate in both directions several times. The big toe, of course, is the main center of attraction, but the little toes can be rotated as well. In general, use the fingers of the right hand for rotating the toes of the right foot and so forth. If the toe catches, clicks, or technique application is painful, try another technique. In evaluating the application of the technique, consider the ease of movement of the toe and any catch or click, resistance to movement.

Lung Press

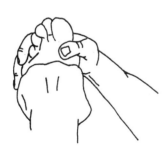

The art in this dessert is the finesse with which the two hands work together to create movement between the bones that form the ball of the foot. Make a fist. For the right foot use the left hand for the fist. Place the flats of the finger on the ball of the foot. Place the right hand on top of the foot. Position it to counter the movement of the left hand.

Press in with the fist against the foot, using the right hand as a backstop. Lessen your pressure and squeeze the foot with your right hand, pushing the foot toward the fist. Now the fist is the backstop. Push with the fist. Push and squeeze with the right hand. A series of four or five sequences completes the dessert.

A smooth wavelike motion is created by coordinating the movements of the two hands. Think of the ebb and flow of a wave. One hand pushes and the other hand responds. Neither hand leaves the foot. Neither hand totally lets up pressure.

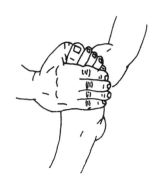

To work the left foot, reverse hands. You can use opposite hands if a sensitive bunion creates a situation where you cannot grasp the foot.

In evaluating the application of technique, consider the give-and-take movement of the ball of the foot. When you push in on the foot, can you feel some flexibility or do you meet resistance?

Spinal Twist

This is a delightful tension reducer. Place your hands around the foot so that the index fingers and thumbs are right next to each other. Position the hands so that the thumbs are on the bottom of the foot and the fingers grip the foot on top. Your hands should now be positioned so that, while index fingers and thumbs are touching, the foot is being gripped on the inside, or arch side.

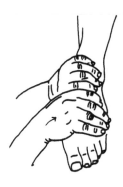

Now turn the hand nearest the toes while keeping the other in a fixed position. Make a back-and-forth motion with the turning hand (imagine a wringing motion with one hand doing all the turning). Maintain an evenly distributed gripping pressure, just enough to hold the foot without letting the hands slip.

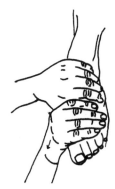

To apply this dessert to the foot, begin at the lower spine reflex area. Make several turns of the hand nearest the toes, keeping the other hand in position. Then reposition **both** hands slightly closer to the toes and repeat. Continue in this manner (i. e., grip and twist, reposition, grip and twist, reposition, etc.) until the index finger of the twisting hand reaches the base of the toes. Do not go into the toe area. Twist both hands at the same time. The attempt is to twist the foot around the spine reflex area (see foot chart), not to impart a wringing sensation to the whole foot. In evaluating the application of technique, consider the ease with which the foot turns and any resistance to turning.

Metatarsal Mover

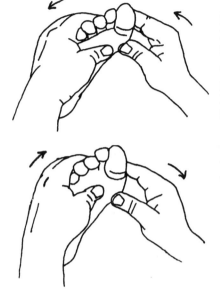

The goal of technique application is to create movement between the metatarsal bones. Grasp the foot as shown. The right hand holds one metatarsal bone and the left hand holds the neighboring metatarsal. Both hands play an equal working role. The flats of the thumbs and fingers are the points of contact with the foot. To practice the technique move the right hand away from you and the left hand toward you. Create a rapid, rhythmic movement of your hands. Repeat with the other metatarsal bones.

In evaluating the application of technique, consider the ease with which you can move the foot. Do you meet some resistance? Is the foot immovable?

The Feathering Touch

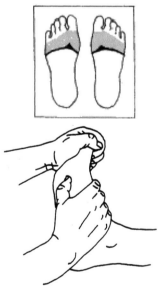

This dessert is particularly effective when applied to the solar plexus/diaphragm reflex area on the bottom of the foot. But it can also be used on the toes (neck, head/sinus) and lymphatic/groin reflex area. Essentially the *feathering touch* describes itself very well. It is a light, rhythmic motion using the *thumb walking* technique. The basic idea is to walk very lightly and rapidly through the reflex area to be *feathered*.

To *feather* the solar plexus/diaphragm reflex area, do not try to hit the reflex points per se. Cover the entire reflex area by starting down in the solar plexus region and *feathering* up through the lung reflex area. Do not concern yourself with the troughs. Work lightly and smoothly, repeatedly walking through the entire region from bottom to top. Since this reflex area is the main storage center for stress in the body, the effect of this dessert should be immediately apparent on the face of your subject. Watch his/her expressions to find the reflex areas or *feathering* techniques which are most pleasing.

Working the Foot

The Big Toe

pituitary
brain
thyroid / parathyroid

seventh cervical

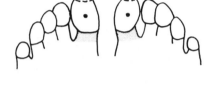

The big toe includes several important reflex areas. Each toe represents half of the head reflex area and contains all five zones. The head joins onto the body just as the toe joins the foot. The important connector between the toe and the foot then corresponds to the neck.

The **pituitary** is an exact pinpoint reflex area. Locating the pituitary reflex point requires measuring the big toe. Since big toes vary in shape and dimensions, it is important to use this measurement procedure. Look for the widest point on either side of the toe. Draw an imaginary line between these points. (See Illus.) In some cases the widest point may be calloused. If the widest point is a callous, use it for your measurement. The pituitary lies on the midpoint of this line. Some lines will be straight across; some will be slanted.

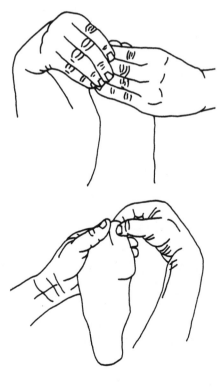

To work the point, you must support and protect your subject's big toe with the holding hand. This prevents excessive bending and pinching of the toe. Place the fingers of the working hand on those of the opposite hand. (See Illus.) Place the thumb just beyond the pituitary point. Use the *hook and back up* technique and be sure to use the corner of the thumb.

Leverage is very important here. Your right hand is the working hand on your subject's right big toe and so forth. This allows the fingers to provide the maximum leverage.

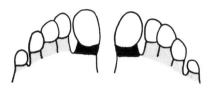

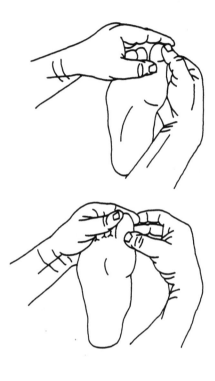

The **thyroid/parathyroid** reflex areas are located above the base of the neck reflex area on the toe. They are, therefore, located at the base of the big toe and of all the other toes. For the moment, we will discuss the technique for working this reflex area on the big toe.

To work the thyroid/parathyroid reflex area, support and protect the toe with the holding hand. Use the thumb to hold the toe to provide a stationary target. Place the fingers of the working hand on those of the holding hand (as shown). Walk across the area using the *thumb walking* technique. Make at least two passes, one high and one low. Several passes are necessary in order to cover the thyroid's wide reflex area. Change hands and walk from the other direction. By working this and the seventh cervical reflex area, you will have covered the entire base of the big toe.

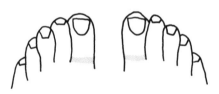

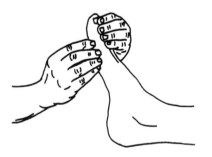

The **seventh cervical** affects everything from the neck to the fingertips. Numbness in the fingers can often be traced to the seventh cervical. To work the seventh cervical, start by anchoring the big toe with the fingertips and thumb. Place the thumb in a comfortable position on the bottom of the foot. Walk forward with the finger around the base of the top of the big toe. Angle the finger. Notice that you have walked around a groove at the base of the toe. An angled finger will fit into this area better than a thumb. (See Illus.)

The Tips of the Toes: Technique Variation

head

brain

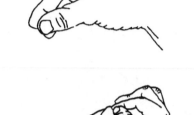

The tips of the toes represent the top of the head. Working this reflex area can have special significance for head problems such as stroke, brain injury, and some eye and ear disorders. The big toe itself represents half of the head and is thus a focal point for this technique. The small toes can be worked in exactly the same way, however.

Anchor the big toe with the thumb and index finger of the holding hand. Either hand can be used. (See Illus.) Join the thumb and index finger of the working hand (as shown). Using the thumb as a support, roll the end of the index finger across a portion of the tip of the toe. The finger actually stays in place while you roll it from one side to the other, exerting a downward pressure.

Reposition the index finger and repeat. Cover the whole tip of the big toe in this manner. Repeat this procedure for the small toes. If you encounter sensitivity, take note. It is a guide to you for locating reflex areas that will need special attention.

The Toes: Thumb Walking

head / brain / sinuses

jaw / teeth / gums

neck / thyroid / throat

The small toes represent a breakdown of the big toe. They are in zones 2, 3, 4, and 5, respectively. The small toes are the fine tuning of the big toe.

The goal of this technique is to walk the thumb down the center and two sidepaths of each toe. There is a natural way that the thumb fits against the toes.

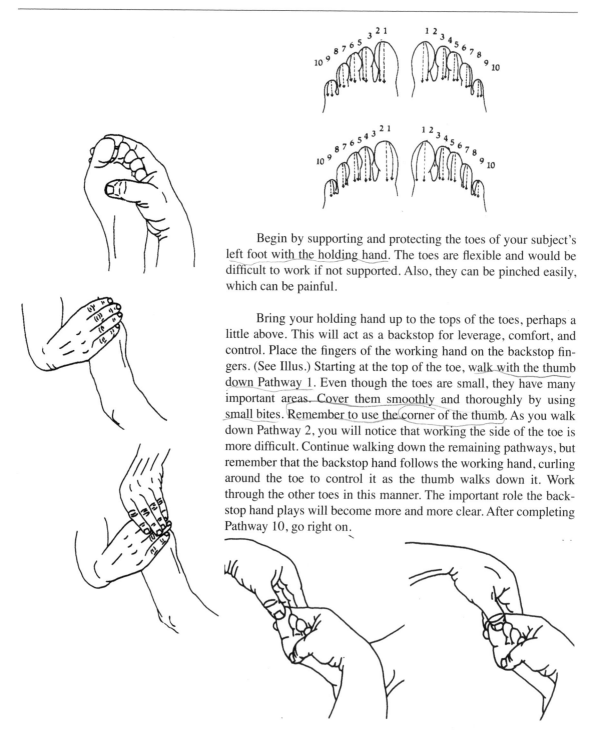

Begin by supporting and protecting the toes of your subject's left foot with the holding hand. The toes are flexible and would be difficult to work if not supported. Also, they can be pinched easily, which can be painful.

Bring your holding hand up to the tops of the toes, perhaps a little above. This will act as a backstop for leverage, comfort, and control. Place the fingers of the working hand on the backstop fingers. (See Illus.) Starting at the top of the toe, walk with the thumb down Pathway 1. Even though the toes are small, they have many important areas. Cover them smoothly and thoroughly by using small bites. Remember to use the corner of the thumb. As you walk down Pathway 2, you will notice that working the side of the toe is more difficult. Continue walking down the remaining pathways, but remember that the backstop hand follows the working hand, curling around the toe to control it as the thumb walks down it. Work through the other toes in this manner. The important role the backstop hand plays will become more and more clear. After completing Pathway 10, go right on.

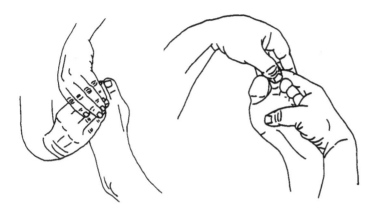

You are still working on the right foot. Change hands and follow the same method to walk down the bottoms of the toes. Remember to curl the holding fingers to control the toes. Follow the same procedure for working the small toes of the left foot.

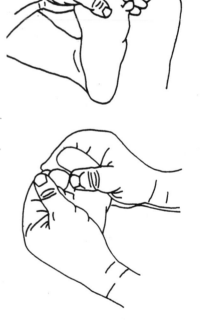

To finish working the bottoms and sidepaths, walk up them the same way you walked *down* them. Use the thumb to walk from the base of each toe up each sidepath to the top of the toe. Then walk up the bottom of each toe from the base to the top. Change hands and work the other sidepaths and bottoms again (as shown). This part of the technique is beneficial for various problems in the head and neck reflex areas, particularly those in the neck muscles, which are prime candidates for storing tension and stress.

Note: This technique may not be possible with short or tightly curled toes. The sidepaths, however, can usually be covered on any toe, no matter how curled.

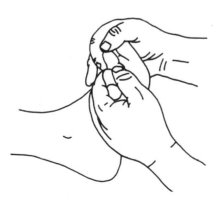

The Toes: Finger Walking

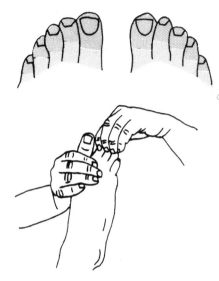

To complete the coverage of the small toes, the tops of each toe must be worked. The sidepaths and tops of the small toes are worked using the *finger walking* technique. If your subject complains of shoulder problems, it may be helpful to walk down into the lung reflex area on the top of the foot as you work from the tops of each toe.

Use the thumb of the holding hand as a brace on the toe you work. Starting at the top of the toe, walk the finger down the top sidepath and top center of each toe. Switch hands and cover the other top sidepaths.

This technique will help you explore a variety of problems in the head-neck region. These include lymph gland and shoulder problems and tension. When using this technique, be careful not to stretch or hurt the sensitive skin between the toes.

The Ridge Along the Base of the Toes: Thumb Walking

eye / ear

tops of shoulders

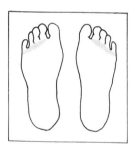

The object of this technique is to walk with the thumb along the ridge at the base of the toes. To maximize effectiveness, the flesh in this area must be thinned out.

With the holding hand, pull the pad of the foot down to thin out this flesh (as shown). This opens the area up. Do not squeeze the foot, because that would put more flesh between you and those reflexes. Do not hold the toes back either, for that would tighten the skin, making it even more difficult to work the area.

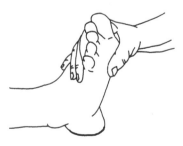

Using the thumb, walk along the top of this ridge. Exert the pressure downward (toward the heel) along the top of the ridge. Do not walk against the toes or you will miss the reflexes. Change hands and walk across the ridge from the opposite direction. Walking from both directions ensures hitting all points.

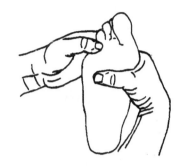

On the feet, the eye and the ear reflex areas overlap. Anatomically, the inner ear is behind the eye. So on the foot, the inner ear reflex area is on the ridge between the third and fourth toes.

Note: In general, the foot follows a logical pattern relating the anatomy of the body to reflex areas on the feet. The location of the eye/ear reflex area seems to be an exception. Even though the reflexes of the eyes and ears are probably located in the toes themselves, this part of the foot represents the muscles on the tops of the shoulders, which support the head and neck. The cranial nerves that provide innervation to the eyes and ears emerge from under the skull into the neck muscles.

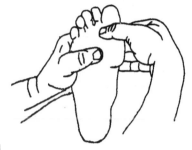

Solar Plexus / Diaphragm Reflex Area on the Bottom of the Foot: Thumb Walking

If one had to choose only one reflex area on the foot to work, it would have to be this one. This reflex area is the body's midbrain, a nerve network with connections to all parts of the trunk and limbs. This is the primary target reflex area for releasing tension and relaxing your subject. (See Illus.)

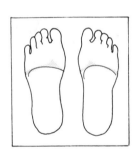

The thumb walking technique is used to work the reflex area. On the right foot, hold the toes back with the left hand. Place the fingers of the working hand on top of the foot for leverage. Walk through the reflex area with the thumb. Try it from several directions. Pay particular attention to the trough below the ball of the foot in line with the big toe. (See Illus.) Frequently, your subject will have stored a great amount of tension in this reflex area. It is also associated with a hiatal hernia, a hernia of part of the stomach into the opening in the diaphragm. This reflex area on the left foot is usually more tender because the hernia is prone to occur more on the left side of the diaphragm. To work the left foot, reverse hands and repeat the procedure.

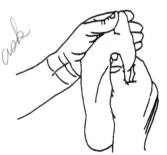

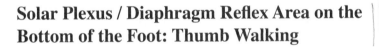

47

Introduction to the Lung Reflex Area

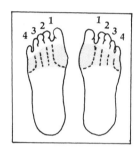

Reflexes pass through the foot. What this means is that the reflex areas listed as being on top of the foot can be worked from the bottom too. This does not mean that there is a "top of the lung" or a "bottom of the lung" reflex area on the foot. Frequently it will prove easier to work these reflex areas on the top of the foot because there is little flesh to inhibit your hitting the points.

Lung Reflex Area on the Bottom of the Foot: Thumb Walking

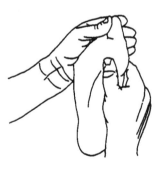

chest

lung

heart

breast

shoulder

The picture of the body at the left is flat. But your body is three-dimensional. Imagine for a moment that this section is isolated from the rest of the body. On the front of it would be the shoulder, chest, and breast. On the back are the shoulder, shoulder blades, and the reflex areas in between. Sandwiched between are the lungs and the heart. When you work the lung reflex area on the bottom of the foot, you touch all of these reflex areas. The whole reflex area extends from the base of the toes through the ball of the foot. (See Illus.)

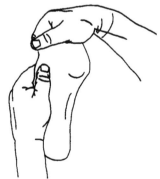

To work the lung reflex area on the bottom of the right foot, hold the toes back with the left hand. This permits you to walk up the four troughs between the toes on the ball of the foot. Use the thumb to walk around the curved portion and up Trough 1. (See Illus.) The starting point for this is actually the diaphragm/solar plexus. Do not worry about working both sides of the trough. Use the same thumb to walk up Trough 2.

Change hands (the thumb is more efficient if not stretched too far). Hold the toes back with the right hand. Walk up Trough 3 with the thumb of the left hand. Use the same hand to walk around the curve and up Trough 4. This is the shoulder reflex area.

To work the left foot, follow the same procedure. The right hand is now the holding hand. When walking through Trough 1 on the left foot, one problem that may show up is a hiatal hernia, a ballooning of the esophagus through a weakened wall of the diaphragm. In this case, both feet will be tender in Trough 1, but the left foot will be more sensitive.

Lung Area and Below on the Top of the Foot: Finger Walking

chest / breast

lung

shoulder

upper back

lymphatic drain

The object here is to work both sides of each of the four troughs on the top of each foot. These troughs are deep, so part of this technique involves exposing them through proper foot holding.

Refer to the illustrations. Beginning with the left foot, use the right hand as the holding hand. The index finger of the left hand does the walking. There are three important parts to this technique:

First, widen the troughs and make them easier to see and work by spreading the toes apart. To do this, place two fingers of the holding hand (as shown) for stability. The thumb does the spreading.

Second., to open the reflex area while providing a stationary object to work, push on the ball of the foot with the flat of the thumb of the working hand. Experiment in pushing the thumb on the ball of the foot and watch how it exposes the troughs on top of the foot.

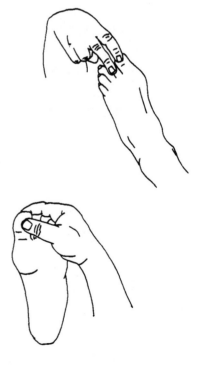

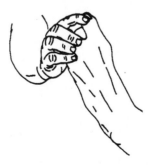

Left foot
- hiatal hernia, a ballooning of the esophagus through a weakened wall of the diaphragm may show

49

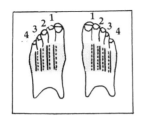

Third, with the index finger of the working hand, walk down Trough 1 to the waistline. The left-hand finger will do best on the left side of the troughs (your left). Use the index finger of the right hand for the right side of the troughs. Using the correct finger ensures that optimum leverage will be attained.

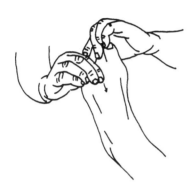

Work the rest of the troughs in the same manner. When you work the right side of the troughs, the left hand is the holding hand. The *finger walking* is especially critical in this technique. Any extra bending or unbending motion can cause nail marks or dragging of the tender skin on top of the foot.

The walking motion must always be forward with a constant, steady pressure. The temptation is to hit the point by drawing back across it. This would cause pain or irritation. It is not a good way to hit the points. Rocking the finger too far with on-off-on-off pressure will leave a trail of fingernail marks on the foot. This is unnecessary.

The walking finger should be angled slightly. In addition to opening up the reflex area, pushing up firmly with the thumb on the ball of the foot provides leverage for the walking finger.

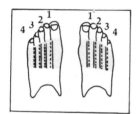

Wide feet can be difficult in this technique. It may be too difficult to stretch the hand around the toes to walk down the troughs. Try walking down one side of Trough 2. Then change your angle and walk down the other side. Do the first two troughs this way.

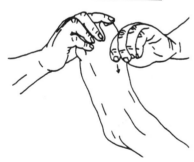

The finger walking technique for the top of the foot takes practice. Spreading the toes, pushing with the thumb on the ball of the foot, and walking with the finger are all equally important to a successful technique. When done properly, the technique is comfortable and effective.

A variation on this technique is to use the finger walking technique to walk across the troughs below the base of the toes.

Waistline Area and Above on the Bottom of the Foot: Thumb Walking

Right Foot / Left foot

adrenal gland / adrenal gland

liver and gallbladder / spleen

stomach (part) / stomach

pancreas (part) / pancreas

kidney (top of) / kidney (top of)

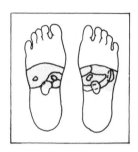

As you can see from the list above, many vital organs are represented in this section of the foot. The thumb walking technique is used to work all of these reflexes in a systematic way. For maximum effectiveness it is necessary to be conscious of the specific organ's reflex location.

The region is bounded by the diaphragm and the waistline. (See Illus.) On the foot, the diaphragm reflex area is defined by the lower border of the ball of the foot. The waistline is an imaginary line drawn across the foot from the fifth metatarsal, which is the protruding bone midway down the outside of the foot. Find this bone on your own foot. Then draw a line from the high spot on this bone straight across the foot. This is your waistline.

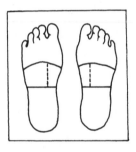

Another locator is the tendon. It assists you in locating the adrenal glands and the kidney reflex areas. In the body, the adrenal glands sit on top of the kidneys. Both kidneys, however, are tilted. This causes the adrenal glands to lie on the inside of the tendon, with the kidneys on the outside.

Look at your foot once again. Flex the toes. Notice that when you pull the toes back, a rather thick tendon protrudes, running from the big toe back to the heel. If you have a thick foot, you may have to feel for it. The adrenal glands' reflex areas lie on the inside of this tendon, halfway up the waistline to the diaphragm. All of the other vital organs can be located within the waistline-diaphragm-adrenal boundary.

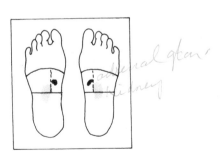

51

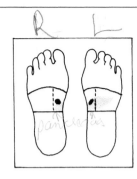

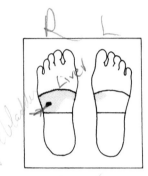

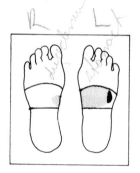

The pancreas fits below the adrenal gland, with a slight upward slant. The majority of the pancreas reflex area is on the left foot, but remember to work the small portion of it on the right foot.

The liver/gallbladder is a rather large reflex area under the diaphragm line. It extends from the outside of the right foot all the way across to the left foot. The gallbladder is located on the right foot but may vary a bit in location.

The spleen is positioned under the diaphragm line on the left foot. Much smaller than the liver, it is locate at the tail end of the pancreas.

The stomach lies mostly on the left foot, overlapping several reflex areas. The duodenum, the prime candidate for ulceration, lies on the right foot, just to the outside edge of the pancreas.

Slightly above the waistline on both feet are parts of the kidney and large colon. The kidneys are positioned along the waistline, with the left kidney slightly higher. When working this reflex area on the outside of the tendon, you encounter the top half of each kidney.

Parts of the large intestine run through this reflex area. Working the large intestine, however, is discussed in the section on the waistline and below (page 48).

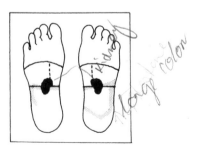

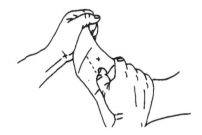

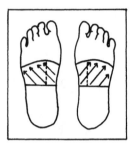

There is a suggested order to working these reflex areas on the feet. On the right foot, use the left hand to hold. Walk in to pinpoint the pancreas. Starting at the waistline on the inside of the foot tendon, walk with the thumb along the tendon until you locate the reflex area of the adrenal glands. Then work diagonally across this reflex area, letting up on the tendon as needed. Change hands and walk the other thumb diagonally through the reflex area. Make several passes. But set up some kind of pattern for yourself so that you do not miss even the smallest part of the reflex area. You should be working the entire waistline-to-diaphragm area at this point. Cover it thoroughly. Repeat the procedure for the left foot.

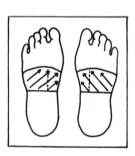

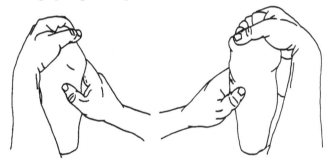

The Arm Area on the Outside of the Foot: Thumb and Finger Walking

arm

elbow

hand

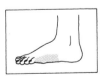

The arm reflex area runs from the base of the little toe to the fifth metatarsal bone along the outside edge of the foot. In reflex terms this means that it runs from the neck reflex area to the waistline off the shoulder, as the arm does on the body. The reflex area between the neck and the diaphragm generally corresponds to the upper arm; between the diaphragm and waistline (and even into the knee/ leg reflex area) corresponds to the elbow/forearm/ hand.

53

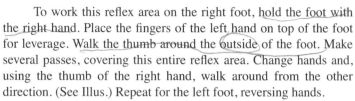

To work this reflex area on the right foot, hold the foot with the right hand. Place the fingers of the left hand on top of the foot for leverage. Walk the thumb around the outside of the foot. Make several passes, covering this entire reflex area. Change hands and, using the thumb of the right hand, walk around from the other direction. (See Illus.) Repeat for the left foot, reversing hands.

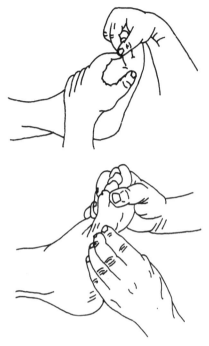

Note: Although it is possible to work the reflex area by walking the thumb up and down the edge of the foot, it is somewhat more difficult because the foot is harder to hold comfortably.

For fine tuning, walk the fingers (index and/or third) through the same reflex area. Do so by first holding the right foot in the right hand, placing the thumb of the left hand on the bottom of the foot for leverage. Once again, make several passes in order to cover the whole reflex area. In this instance, the fingers may have an advantage by enabling you to search out the nooks and crannies of the bones in this reflex area, especially those of the fifth metatarsal. To walk the fingers through this reflex area on the left foot, reverse hands and repeat the procedure.

Below the Waistline on the Bottom of the Foot: Thumb Walking

Right Foot / Left Foot

colon / colon

ileocecal valve / sigmoid colon

small intestine / small intestine

kidney / kidney

lower back/hip/pelvis / lower back/hip/pelvis

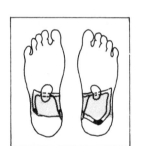

On the right foot this reflex area includes the kidney, half of the small intestine framed by the colon, and the ileocecal valve. The ileocecal valve, which is located at the beginning of the colon, is worked by *pinpointing*. The rest of the reflex area is crisscrossed using the *thumb walking* technique.

Begin by locating the ileocecal valve. It lies between the small and the large intestine reflex areas. This reflex area of the colon around the valve is responsible for the elimination of mucus. If it is not doing its job properly, the mucus is absorbed into the bloodstream and makes its way to other parts of the body. The

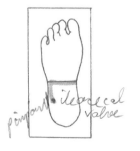

sinuses are a likely spot. For a sinus problem, as well as any mucus problem, the ileocecal valve is an important reflex area to work.

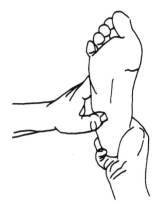

Look at the right foot. Try to visualize the intestines superimposed on it. The waistline bone, the fifth metatarsal, is a helpful reference point. Find the bone and the waistline. The transverse colon runs along this line. Starting at the fifth metatarsal, the ascending colon runs along the foot toward the heel.

To find the ileocecal valve reflex point, run your hand down the outside of the foot from the fifth metatarsal bone to the heel. Do you feel the hollow spot along here? It is in the deepest part of this hollow that the valve is located. (See Illus.) Hook into this spot and back across it with your thumb. Once again, the fingers provide the all-important leverage. It may be difficult at first to break through the reflex area, so walk through it with the thumb from several directions.

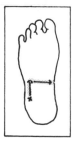 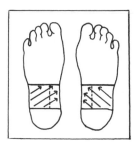 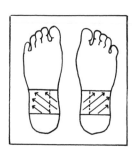

Proceed from the ileocecal to the colon reflex area. Use the thumb of the left hand to walk up the ascending colon to the transverse colon. To work the small intestine reflex area, start by holding the foot back with the right hand. Walk diagonally with the thumb of the left hand across this reflex area, letting up on the tendon as needed. Change hands and work a diagonal pattern. You should be ending your passes in the colon area. This gives you a chance to work the colon from another direction. To complete working this reflex area, walk with your thumb through the kidney reflex area. It sits along the waistline on the outside of the tendon. Connecting into the kidneys are the ureter tubes, whose reflex area continues down into the bladder reflex area at the beginning of the heel.

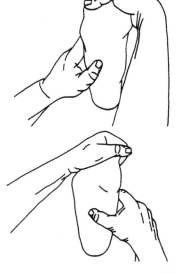

Since we have already walked through much of the kidney reflex area when we crisscrossed the above-the-waist section, it is important not to assume the kidney reflex areas have been completely worked. They are important enough to be walked through from several directions. So hold the foot back with your right hand and walk up the outside of the tendon.

55

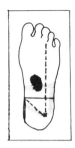

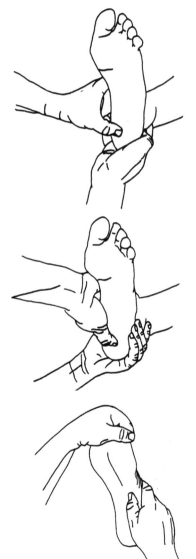

On the left foot, the kidney reflex area and the other half of the colon and small intestine reflex areas are included in the reflex area to be worked. Of special interest is a very important part of the colon, the sigmoid. This S-shaped section of the colon is the last turn before the wastes empty into the rectum for disposal. Because of its position, gas can become trapped here.

First, get an idea of its location. Draw a line on the bottom of the foot across the front edge of the heel (arch). Then draw another line along the inside edge of the heel, also on the bottom of the foot. This should intersect the first line (see Illus.) and form the corner of a box. From this corner, draw a line across the bottom of the heel itself at a 45° angle. The deepest part of the curve in the sigmoid colon is located three to three and one-half zones in from this corner along the 45° line.

There are two ways to work this point. (See Illus.) Choose the one that works best for you. You can use either thumb to walk down the 45° angle. Use the *hook and back up* technique to pinpoint the reflex area. If anchored properly, a great deal of pressure can be applied. Leverage is the key to penetrating this point. If the hand is anchored properly, you can pull with the leverage fingers as the thumb hooks. This is the most difficult point on the foot to reach. The heel may be very tough. It may require several passes from different directions of thumb walking just to loosen it up.

To work the colon reflex areas of the left foot, use the thumb of the right hand to walk up the descending colon and across the transverse colon. Work the small intestine and kidney reflex areas just as you did on the right foot.

Below the Waistline on the Top and Sides of the Feet: Thumb Walking / Finger Walking / Rotating on a Point

hip / sciatic

hip region

tailbone and spine

lymphatic / groin

hip joint (knee / leg)

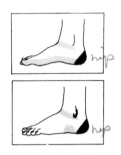

This section of the foot contains reflex areas related to a host of health problems. Included among these are lower back, hip, and tailbone disorders. Internal organs may be affected, such as problems with the colon or the reproductive organs. An injury to the tailbone can cause headaches (including migraines).

To understand how this reflex area of the body corresponds to the feet, it is necessary to transpose the three-dimensional structure of the body to this particular portion of the foot. The spine is on the backside. The hip bone meets the spine and wraps around to the front of the body. What this means is that the top and sides of the feet contain important reflex areas directly related to this three-dimensional view of the lower back reflex area of the body. This is a large reflex area. You must use several different techniques to work it. The goal is to hit every single part of the reflex area.

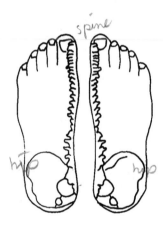

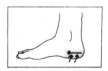

The tailbone / rectum / lower spine region is an area of the body prone to injury and stress. Often, injuries to the tailbone can be traced to childhood. Such injuries will make the corresponding reflex area of the foot extremely sensitive. The reflex areas to be worked run along the inside of the foot, below the waistline, well into the heel. (See Illus.)

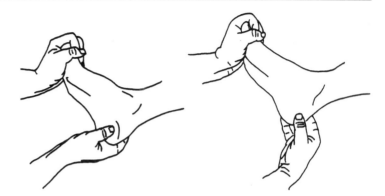

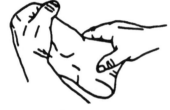

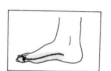

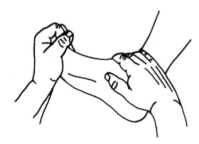

To work the tailbone reflex area, cup the heel of the right foot in the left hand. Walk in a crisscross pattern through the reflex area with the thumb of the right hand. Make several passes. In general, walk from the bottom of the heel upwards. Change the angle and try to cover the reflex area thoroughly. Now, walk from the bottom of the heel upwards. Change the angle and try to cover the reflex area thoroughly. Be patient and persistent. To work the lower spine, simply walk the thumb up along the spine reflex area from the tailbone region. Pivot the working hand to maintain good leverage.

Continue walking with the thumb along the entire length of the spine reflex area. Since the reflex area of the spine between the lower back region and the seventh cervical is a wide, general area (see Illus.), use the *thumb walking* technique from several directions.

You can also use one or two fingers to walk around from the bottom through this region to the top of the foot (as shown). Repeat this procedure on the left foot, changing hands accordingly.

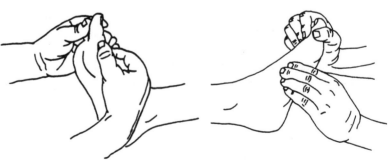

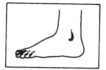

The region around the outside ankle bone is the prime target when dealing with any hip or sciatic problem. Use the *finger walking* technique to walk around this reflex area. The thumb is too awkward and difficult to control in this reflex area.

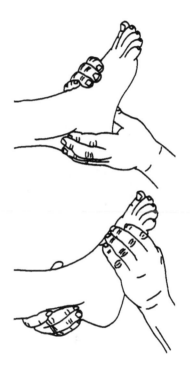

Begin by cupping the right foot in your left hand. Use the index or third finger of the left hand to walk up through this reflex area. Walk around the back of the ankle bone several times. When walking around the ankle bone, walk in the crease around it. If you walk short of this crease, you'll hit the Achilles tendon. If you overrun it. you'll be hitting the ankle bone itself.

To complete the hip/sciatic reflex area on the right foot, cup the right hand under the ankle and heel. Walk with the index or third finger of the left hand from the top of the foot down around the ankle bone. (See Illus.) Be sure to hit the crease. Walking from the top of the foot down to the bottom of the ankle bone gives the deepest penetration.

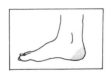 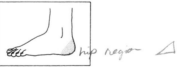

hip region

The hip region is often involved in lower back problems. (See Illus.) The reflex areas are found on the inside and outside of the foot. They are triangular in shape and are worked using the *finger walking* technique. To work these reflex areas, cup the working hand around the back of the ankle. This provides leverage for the walking fingers. Walk down the reflex area, making several passes.

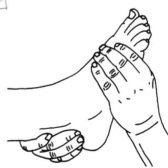

59

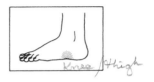

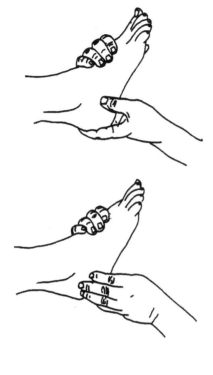

The reflex area of the foot that actually corresponds to the hip joint has also been successfully worked for knee/thigh problems. These reflex areas are linked by the muscles which originate around the hip bone and attach to the leg, including the knee. On the foot, the reflex area is bounded by the fifth metatarsal, the front edge of the heel on the bottom, and the bony area on the side of the foot.

Use either the *thumb* or *finger walking* technique to work the reflex area. No particular precaution need be taken to hold the foot. Just keep the foot stationary. To use the thumb, plant the finger on the opposite side of the foot for leverage. Make several passes. Similarly, to walk with the finger through this reflex area, plant the thumb on the bottom of the foot for leverage (as shown). Again, make several passes.

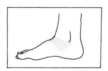 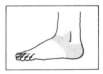

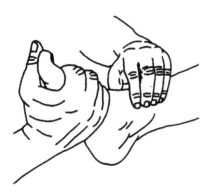

Rotating on a point is used to work the areas corresponding to the lower back region. Begin by *pinpointing* in the areas described above. (See Illus.) Notice that this is a bony region. The goal is to search the nooks and crannies of this region for tender points. When you find a sensitive point, exert pressure on it with the index finger. You can use other combinations of fingers, but the index finger is able to exert the best pressure because of its ideal opposition to the thumb, the leverage giver.

Once you have located a sensitive point, apply the finger pressure. With the holding hand, grasp the foot below the base of the big toe on the inside of the foot. Rotate the foot with the holding hand. This will give a sense of increased pressure at the tender point. Shift the pressure finger around the region, exploring for other sensitive points. Rotate the foot in both directions at least five times. Do not dig with the fingernail. Of course, it is a good idea to keep your nails short enough to prevent any significant nail/skin contact. This technique is ideal for working on your own feet as well. If you wish, you can rotate your foot at the ankle without the aid of a holding hand. Just *pinpoint* the sore spots and turn the ankle in both directions. Variation: Multiple finger walking technique.

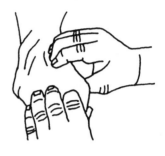

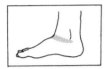 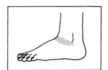

Most of the lymphatic nodes in the body are located in the groin, armpits, and neck. Clustered in these locations, they protect the internal organs from infections in the extremities. All five zones on both feet are affected by each of the three lymphatic reflex areas. The region around the ankle encompasses all five zones and has been found to be effective in working on problems in any of the lymph glands. Included are the groin and the fallopian tubes.

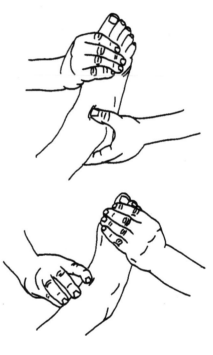

The reflex area to be worked runs from the inside of the ankle bone around the top of the foot (crease) to the outside of the ankle bone. (See Illus.) This crease can be worked as a wide area by making several passes. Particular emphasis must be given to the primary reflex area (as shown). To work with the thumb, hold the foot upright and stationary. Wrap the fingers of the working hand around the ankle and walk with the thumb along the crease. Change hands and walk with the other thumb from the opposite direction. To walk with the index finger (optional), use the same principles, using the thumb for leverage. You can also try walking both index fingers at the same time by placing the thumbs of both hands on the bottom of the foot and walking up on both sides until the two fingers meet in the middle, on the top of the foot.

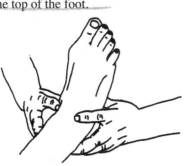

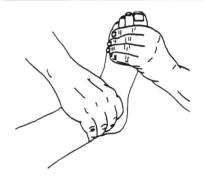

Swelling frequently affects this region because of lymph system problems. A little finesse can be applied when the reflex area is sensitive to the touch. A *dessert* (see Illus.) can allow you to work the reflex area in spite of the tenderness. Bridge your hand over the crease, fitting the thumb and first finger into the crease itself. Rotate the foot in both directions at least five times. (Generally the left hand works better bridging the right foot, etc.) You can also use the *rotating on a point* technique in the lymph reflex area to locate and work sore points within it.

To work the left foot, repeat the above procedure exactly. Reverse hands when appropriate.

Variation: Multiple finger walking technique.

Reproductive System on the Sides of the Heel: Pinpointing

uterus / prostate

ovary / testicle

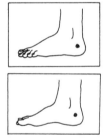

The uterus/prostate reflex area is located on the inside of the foot below the ankle bone. It is a pinpoint reflex area, so correctly locating it is crucial to hitting the point effectively. This reflex area of the foot is commonly tender, but this does not necessarily mean problems specific to the reproductive organs and glands. Working this reflex area can be helpful, for example, in alleviating allergic reactions.

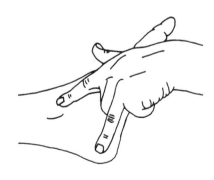

To pinpoint the reflex area, place the tip of the index finger on the ankle bone (inside the foot) and the tip of the fourth finger on the back corner of the heel. Draw the third finger in until it forms a straight line with the others and establishes the midpoint. This is the uterus/prostate reflex area to be worked. (See Illus.)

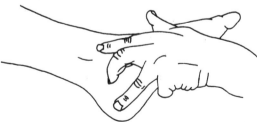

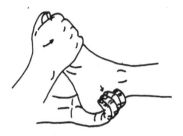

To work the area on the right foot, use the left hand. Cup the heel, curling the third finger in such a way as to place its tip on the point to be worked. The thumb should be positioned in the lymphatic area on the top of the foot. Now rotate the foot with the right hand in both directions several times. You can vary the amount of pressure you use with the third finger as appropriate. By *rotating on a point,* you *pinpoint* accurately while limiting the amount of discomfort for your subject.

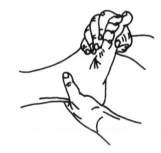

To work the left foot reflex area, simply reverse hands and repeat the procedure.

To locate the ovary/testicle reflex area, use the same technique as you used for the uterus/prostate. (See Illus.) Because the reflex area is on the bone outside of the foot, walk through it with the thumb of the left hand. You can also walk the finger of the right hand through this reflex area, holding the foot just as you do for working the hip/sciatic reflex area.

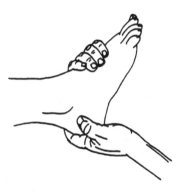

On the left foot, repeat the procedure, reversing hands.

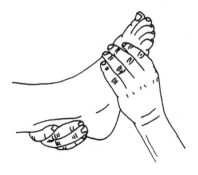

Technique Session Pattern

Practice applying techniques in a repeatable sequence.	**Check foot for cuts, callouses, bruises.**	Side to side	Foot flicking	Rotating the ankle
Spinal twist	Lung press	Solar plexus	Toe rotation	Pituitary
Thyroid	Seventh cervical	Top of head	Side to side	Head/neck/sinus
Eye/ear	Head/neck/sinus	Metatarsal mover	Lung/Chest/Breast	Below Waistline
Lung press	Solar plexus	Heart/left	Lung/Chest/Breast	Shoulder

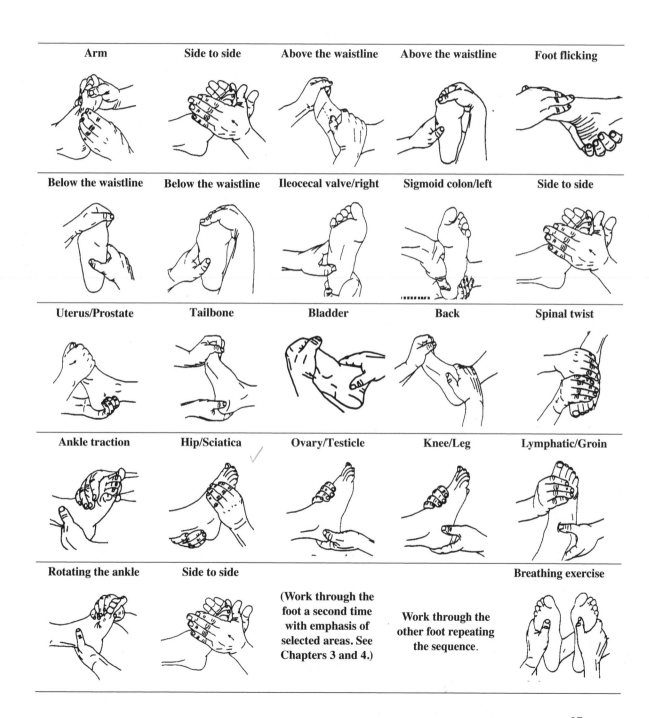

Arm	Side to side	Above the waistline	Above the waistline	Foot flicking
Below the waistline	Below the waistline	Ileocecal valve/right	Sigmoid colon/left	Side to side
Uterus/Prostate	Tailbone	Bladder	Back	Spinal twist
Ankle traction	Hip/Sciatica	Ovary/Testicle	Knee/Leg	Lymphatic/Groin
Rotating the ankle	Side to side	(Work through the foot a second time with emphasis of selected areas. See Chapters 3 and 4.)	Work through the other foot repeating the sequence.	Breathing exercise

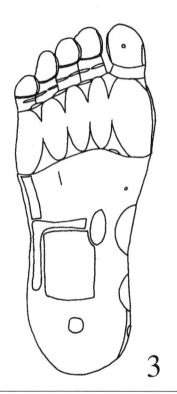

3

Assessing the Foot

Assessing the Foot

Assessing the foot is a skill acquired by the reflexologist to identify areas of the foot for technique application and / or emphasis. From this information, a plan for further work can be created. In addition, a reflexologist's evaluation can be communicated to the client. Assessment also provides the basis for working with medical professionals and health insurance claims. The reflexologist's work with a client is, thus, summed up in reflexological terms for documentation in writing or discussion with other health professionals.

The three-stage process described in this chapter is designed to guide you through an assessment of the stress response of the individual. Assessing the foot is a reading of the stresses the foot and body have experienced. The goal of assessing the foot is to (1) Observe and identify stress cues on the feet that indicate the wear-and-tear patterns; (2) Draw inferences from the stress cues to make an evaluation of the adaptation by the foot and body to stress in the terms of reflexology; and (3) Reach some conclusions about the individual's response to stress.

Observing Stress Cues of the Foot

A key element in assessing the foot is your ability to observe. Observing is a process of asking yourself a series of questions that allow you to evaluate the foot. Questions center around stress cues. *A stress cue is any part of the foot that shows adaptation to stress.* Adaptation to stress is noted through what you observe visibly and with your sense of touch.

Note and measure

Several general rules apply when observing the foot and identifying stress cues. First, observing the foot is a technique of noting and measuring. Noting each stress cue and considering its dimensions provides an opportunity to systematically chronicle the stress pattern of the foot.

Comparing and contrasting is a technique common to identifying any stress cue. The individual's left foot is compared to his or her right foot. The ball of the foot is compared to the arch of the foot. This individual's feet are compared to the feet of others. You can, thus, establish a frame of reference to identify stress cues.

Compare and contrast

Comparing and contrasting is also a part of the questions utilized to identify and evaluate stress cues. For example, when considering the question, "Is this foot puffy?" the answer is "Yes, compared to other feet, it is puffy." Or, "No, compared to other feet, it isn't puffy."

Look for the noteworthy when observing the feet. For example, consider the question, "Which is the most significant, noteworthy characteristic of this particular foot?" Or, consider a question such as, "Is this the thinnest foot I've ever seen?" Or, "Is this the most callousing I've seen on any foot?" If your answer to yourself is yes to any such question, it is a foot with a stress cue to which you will compare future feet and stress cues you will observe. Also, it is a stress cue that can act as a frame of reference for assessment of the individual's foot.

Look for the noteworthy

Take into consideration normal wear and tear when observing any foot. The foot of a sixty-year-old is not the foot of a twenty-year-old. A certain number of stress cues can be expected with the wear and tear of stress over the years. (See "Stress History.") The foot is observed within its context. Observations are made such as, "This foot shows signs of stress adaptation but, all things considered, not as many as I would expect."

Consider normal wear and tear

To practice observing the foot and identifying stress cues, observe a variety of feet. Compare young feet to older feet. Compare men's feet to women's feet. With practice, you will learn to quickly identify stress cues that create targets and target strategies for your technique application.

Observe a variety of feet

We have organized a systematic observation of the foot into four basic techniques: observing visual stress cues, observing touch stress cues, observing sensitivity stress cues, and observing press and assess stress cues. We have selected particular vocabulary words such as puffiness, thickness, and hard tonus to serve as terms to describe stress cues and note gradations of stress.

Observing Visual Stress Cues

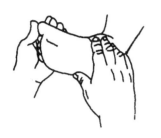

Observing visual signs of stress on the foot involves noting the visible surface of the foot. Just as any landscape has its landmarks, the surface of the foot is notable for its signs of adaptation to stress.

To observe the foot in more detail, begin with the toes and proceed on to the base of the toes, ball of the foot, the arch, the heel, the top, the inside and outside of the foot in a systematic manner.

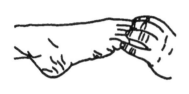

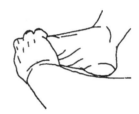

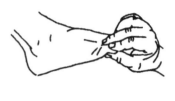

Consider the following commonly found stress cues. Visually observable foot stress is described in terms of texture, foot features, and color. Can you find any of these characteristics of stress on the foot you are observing?

Texture

Texture observations are made to note the surface character of the foot. The goal is to observe any adaptation to stress that appears on the surface of the foot. Texture is described in terms of *puffiness*, *thickness*, and *callousing*.

Observe the foot in general. What is your impression of the foot? Is it a thin foot? A thick foot? Is the surface of the foot consistent in texture? What do you consider the most outstanding visual characteristic of the foot? Do you note several outstanding characteristics? Do the characteristics center around one part of the foot, such as the toes?

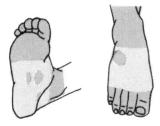

Puffiness
Do you see puffiness on the foot anywhere? Where? How puffy is it? How large is the puffy area? Are there several puffy areas? Is the surface of the foot puffy? Somewhat puffy?

Visual Stress Cues

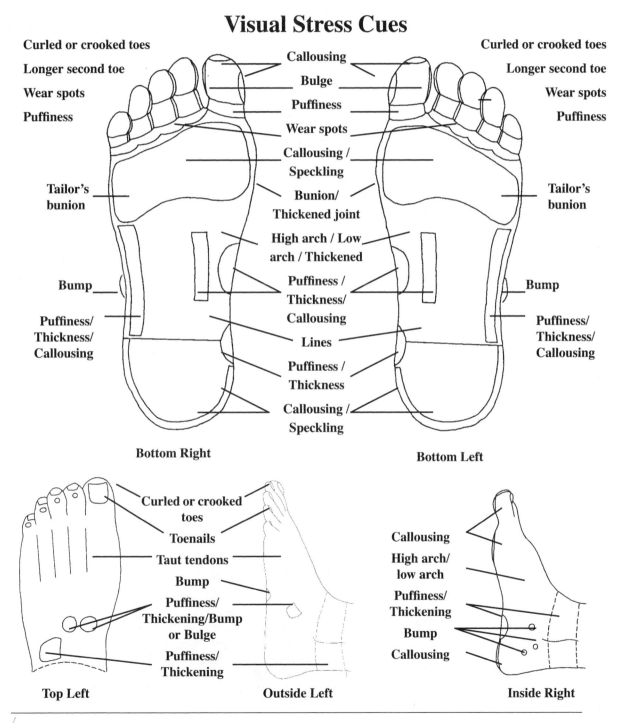

Curled or crooked toes

Longer second toe

Wear spots

Puffiness

Tailor's bunion

Bump

Puffiness/ Thickness/ Callousing

Callousing

Bulge

Puffiness

Wear spots

Callousing / Speckling

Bunion/ Thickened joint

High arch / Low arch / Thickened

Puffiness / Thickness/ Callousing

Lines

Puffiness / Thickness

Callousing / Speckling

Curled or crooked toes

Longer second toe

Wear spots

Puffiness

Tailor's bunion

Bump

Puffiness/ Thickness/ Callousing

Bottom Right

Bottom Left

Curled or crooked toes

Toenails

Taut tendons

Bump

Puffiness/ Thickening/Bump or Bulge

Puffiness/ Thickening

Callousing

High arch/ low arch

Puffiness/ Thickening

Bump

Callousing

Top Left

Outside Left

Inside Right

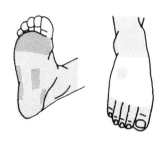

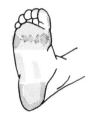

Thickness

Do the feet appear to have areas of thickness or texture that is well-padded and dense? Where? How thick is the area? How large is the thick area? Is the whole foot thick? Somewhat thick?

Callousing

Do you see callousing on the foot anywhere? Where? In several areas? How thick is the callousing? How large is the calloused area? Is the entire bottom of the foot calloused? Are the calluses hard? Clear? Shiny? Yellow? Cracked?

Foot Feature

A foot feature is a distinctive or outstanding visual landmark on the foot. A foot feature indicates a structure of the foot itself that has been altered by adaptation to stress. Several of these stress cues are also considered foot problems.

Observe the foot in general. Do you note any distinctive or outstanding foot features? Are there several foot features? Does both the right and the left foot show the same foot features?

Bunion

Is there a bunion, a protrusion of the joint? How extreme is the bunion? Are all the toes pressed together and/or at an angle to the foot? Is there callousing on or around the bunion? Is the bunion red and inflamed? Are there bunions on both feet?

Visual Stress Cue Observation

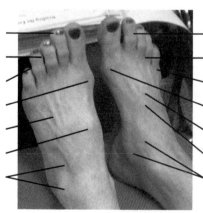

Longer second toe	Longer second toe
Knobby toes	Knobby toes
Toes pressed together	Toes pressed together
Bunion	Bunion
Taut tendons	Taut tendons
Bump	Bump
Bumps and bulges	Bumps and bulges

See p. 227.

Bump or Bulge on top of the foot

Does the foot show pockets of puffiness or thickness formed into bumps or bulges on the tops or sides of the foot? Where? How large an area is involved? Do both feet show the same adaptation to stress?

Corn

Is there a corn on any toe? Several toes? Is the corn hard and clear? Red and inflamed? Do both feet show the same adaptation to stress?

Arch: High, low, lined

How high is the arch of the foot? Is it so high that a wet footprint would show the ball of the foot and heel with little in between? Or, how low is the arch? Is there callousing in the arch of the foot? Does the arch of the foot show lines? Where? Do they radiate from an epi-center? How far across the foot do they extend?

Tailor's bunion

Is there a tailor's bunion, a callousing and/or thickening of the fifth metatarsal head? Do both feet show a tailor's bunion?

Taut tendons

Do taut tendons stand out on the top of the foot?

Visual Stress Cue Observation

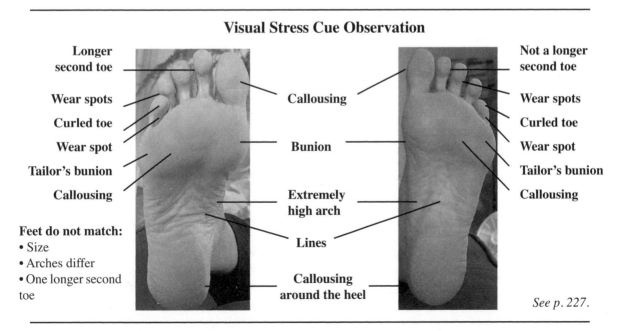

Longer second toe

Wear spots

Curled toe

Wear spot

Tailor's bunion

Callousing

Callousing

Bunion

Extremely high arch

Lines

Callousing around the heel

Not a longer second toe

Wear spots

Curled toe

Wear spot

Tailor's bunion

Callousing

Feet do not match:
• Size
• Arches differ
• One longer second toe

See p. 227.

Toenails

Are any of the toenails thickened, irregularly shaped, etched with lines, yellow, or unusually white in color? Which one(s)? Are there any ingrown nails?

Toes: Curled, crooked, longer second toe, pressed together, wear spots

Are any of the toes curled or crooked? How curled? How crooked? How many are curled or crooked? Are the toe joints knobby in appearance? Do toes on both feet appear curled? To the same extent?

Is the second toe longer than or as long as the big toe? How much longer?

Do the toes show signs of being pressed together? Do all five toes appear to be a single unit or does each toe stand on its own? Do you see wear spots on the bottoms and sides of the toe? How many of the toes show signs of wear spots?

Color

Observing the *color* of the foot is a matter of noting the consistency of skin tone. While color does not necessarily show circulatory stress, color serves as a general indicator of circulation. A very white foot shows a lack of circulation to the foot. A very red foot indicates a lack of circulation from the foot. A blue foot shows a lack of oxygen. White speckling shows an interruption in circulation. Observe the foot. Is the skin tone of the foot natural in color? Is the color of the foot uniform? Is there any white speckling? Where? Over how large an area? Is the whole foot very white? Very red? Cyanotic (blue)?

Observing the Touch Stress Cue

Observing the touch stress cue involves noting the feel of the foot as thumb and finger walking techniques are applied. More than any other stress cue, the cue of touch provides a valuable asset to the reflexologist. When you apply technique to the foot, what do you feel? What you feel, the nature of the foot itself, is directly linked to the stress the foot has experienced. As a rule of thumb, the puffier, the thicker, the harder the tonus, the more adaptation to stress has taken place over time. Also, the pattern of stress is more deeply ingrained as a learning experience, and a longer time period will be required to condition the foot with pressure technique.

Touch Stress Cues

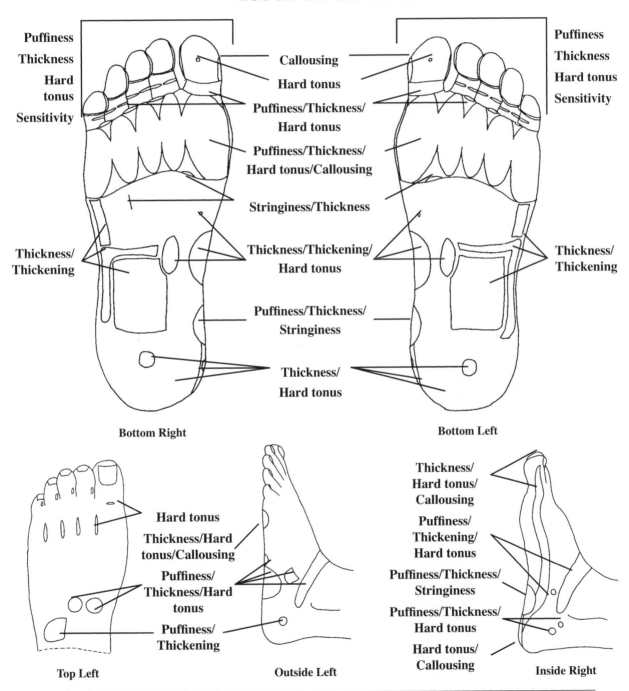

Puffiness
Thickness
Hard
tonus
Sensitivity

Callousing
Hard tonus

Puffiness/Thickness/
Hard tonus

Puffiness/Thickness/
Hard tonus/Callousing

Stringiness/Thickness

Thickness/
Thickening

Thickness/Thickening/
Hard tonus

Puffiness/Thickness/
Stringiness

Thickness/
Hard tonus

Puffiness
Thickness
Hard tonus
Sensitivity

Thickness/
Thickening

Bottom Right

Bottom Left

Hard tonus
Thickness/Hard
tonus/Callousing
Puffiness/
Thickness/Hard
tonus
Puffiness/
Thickening

Top Left

Outside Left

Thickness/
Hard tonus/
Callousing
Puffiness/
Thickening/
Hard tonus
Puffiness/Thickness/
Stringiness
Puffiness/Thickness/
Hard tonus
Hard tonus/
Callousing

Inside Right

75

Tonus: resistance to pressure technique

Touch cues are described in terms of tonus, or the resistance to pressure technique application, as perceived by the reflexologist. *Puffiness*, *thickness*, *hard tonus*, *callousing*, and *stringiness* are terms utilized to note qualities and gradations of the felt surface. Foot temperature evaluation is a further touch assessment technique.

Compare one part of the foot to another

As you work through the foot, compare your touch observations in one part of the foot to the others. For example, does the ball of the foot show the same touch characteristics as the arch of the foot? Then, is the whole foot uniform in its feel? Do both feet show the same touch characteristics?

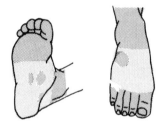

Begin your touch observations with the application of thumb walking technique to the ball of the foot. Go on to apply technique to the toes, the base of the toes, the arch, heel, inside, and outside of the foot. Some of the touch stress cues share the same name as visual stress cues. Be sure to make a touch observation of the visual cues of the same name you have observed. The touch observation is added to your visual observation. As you apply technique to the foot, do you observe any of the following stress cues?

Puffiness
Is there a feeling of puffiness when you apply thumb walking technique to any part of the foot? Does the surface under your thumb feel soft and spongy? Fluidlike? Puffy with some resistance to pressure? Puffy with a stringy band? Where is the puffiness? Over how large an area? The whole foot? How does the puffiness contrast with the surrounding area? Is the surrounding area somewhat puffy? Different in tone?

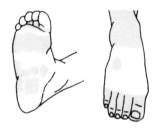

Thickness
Do you feel solid resistance, a thickness, when you apply pressure to any part of the foot? Where? How thick is it? Does it have a distinctive shape? Over how large an area? The whole foot? Does the foot feel somewhat thick all over? When you apply technique to the foot, do you feel a uniformity of thickness?

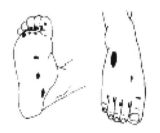

Hard tonus
Do you feel an area of concentrated hardness? Where? Over how large an area? What is the shape of the area? Is the hard tonus surrounded by thick tonus? Puffiness? Callousing? Is there a sharp contrast between the area of hard tonus and the surrounding area?

Do you find a variety of touch stress cues ranging from puffiness to thickening to thickened to hardened?

Callousing

When you apply pressure technique to a calloused part of the foot, what do you feel? Do you feel thickness? Hardness? Is the callousing somewhat hard? Hard with a surrounding area of thickness? How large an area is calloused? Is there a distinctive shape to the callousing? If there are several calloused areas on the foot, are they uniform in callousing?

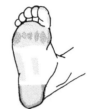

Stringiness

When applying pressure technique to any part of the foot, do you feel stringiness or a resistance to pressure over a stringlike area? Does the stringiness feel like a thin wire or a thick rope?

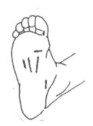

Temperature

What is your initial impression of the foot's temperature? Is the foot hot or cold to the touch initially? Perspiring? (A warmer than usual foot shows an overly active circulatory system. A cooler than usual foot indicates an under-active circulatory system. A perspiring foot shows an over-active elimination system.)

Do both feet show the same or similar touch stress cues? Do both feet show a concentration of touch stress cues in the same parts of the foot, such as the heels?

Observing Sensitivity Stress Cues

A natural part of applying pressure technique to the feet is a response of sensitivity by the client. Although it is your goal to apply technique within the comfort zone of the individual, his or her response of sensitivity provides a stress cue to you. It is a stress cue that calls for immediate evaluation.

If the individual responds to your technique application with a report of sensitivity, ask questions. You want to clarify your image of the sensitive area, and you want to allow the individual to give you feedback. Questions such as, "Is that sensitive?" or "Is that very sensitive?" create an opportunity for the individual to comment. "No, it hurts good" or "Yes, it hurts but go on" is a signal to continue your work with respect for the area. "Yes, it hurts" is a response that calls for avoidance of the area.

Clarify report of sensitivity

Respond to sensitivity

The individual may say something such as, "What's that?" This is a clue that you have found a sensitive area. (Remember that your response should be phrased in the vocabulary of reflexology, such as, "This is what we consider in reflexology theory the ___ reflex area." Typically, the individual will ask a further question such as, "What does it mean?" Again, phrase your response in the vocabulary of reflexology, such as, "We view sensitivity as an indicator of stress in a reflex area, a weak link rather than a problem.")

Consider the sensitivity

In either of the above situations, your evaluation of the sensitivity continues with a comparison of the sensitivity to the other stress cues in the area. What did the sensitive area feel like to you? Are there visual and touch stress cues? How large an area is sensitive? From what you feel, are you surprised at the level of sensitivity or is it about what you would expect considering the foot stress? Does the sensitivity change with the application of technique? Does the area become more sensitive? Less sensitive? Does the sensitivity go away? Is the area too sensitive to touch?

Respect sensitivity

Some individuals are more sensitive than others, and some individuals like a lighter touch in technique application. Remember, sensitivity and the client's preferred level of pressure should always be respected, and techniques should be applied within the individual's comfort range.

A child will respond differently from an adult to technique application. A child's means of communicating his or her opinion about your work is to withdraw the foot or giggle. When asked if an area hurts, a child will often respond, "No, it feels funny."

Observing Press and Assess Stress Cues

Assessing the press and assess cues of foot stress involves noting the appearance of the foot when direct pressure is applied to a stretched foot. An area that changes color notably signifies an area of stress adaptation. Press and assess cues are described in terms of coloration and appearance. The foot is stretched or pressed and then observed for red, white, speckled, or bubbled areas.

Big Toe

To apply the press and assess technique to the big toe, place the big toe in a stretched position. Note any change in surface appearance. Do you see *sheets of white* or *red*? Where? On the ball of the toe? The stem of the toe? Over how large an area?

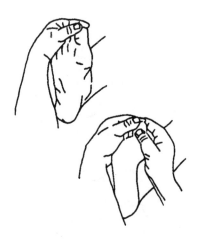

As a further assessment, place the flat of the thumb on the stretched toe and apply direct pressure for several seconds. Lift the thumb and note any change in surface appearance.

Apply thumb walking technique to the area of interest. Reapply the press and assess technique. Does the pattern of color change with ten to fifteen passes of technique? Diminish? Change color?

Ball of Foot

To apply the press and assess technique to the ball of the foot, place the foot in a stretched position. Note any change in the surface appearance of the foot. Do you see *sheets of white, red, white speckling*, or *white bubbling*? Where? Over how large an area?

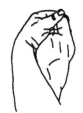

Apply direct pressure to the stretched foot with the flat of the thumb for several seconds. Lift the thumb. Note any change in surface appearance. Do you see areas of red? White? White bubbling? Where? Over how large an area?

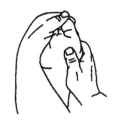

Apply ten to fifteen passes of thumb walking technique to the area of interest. Reapply the press and assess technique. Has the pattern of color changed? Diminished in size?

Arch of the Foot

To apply the press and assess technique to the arch of the foot, place the foot in a stretched position.

Apply direct pressure with the flat of the thumb. Lift the thumb. Observe any changes in color or the appearance of *white speckling* or *bubbling*.

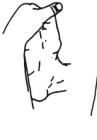
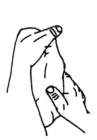

Apply ten to fifteen passes of thumb walking technique to the area of interest. Reapply the press and assess technique. Has the appearance of the foot changed from the previous measurement?

79

Heel

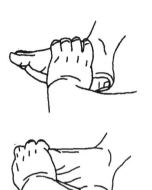

To apply the press and assess technique to the heel, position the thumb so that the edge of the heel is visible.

Apply direct pressure with the flat of the thumb. (To prevent any strain on the thumb from applying pressure to the thick heel, keep the thumb slightly bent.) Observe the area surrounding the pressing thumb. Do you see a noticeable change in color? *White speckling*? *White bubbling*? Where? Over how large an area? Is there a pattern formed? If there is white bubbling, does the bubbling stand out from the foot? Can you feel the raised bubbles?

Lift your thumb. Note the color. Apply ten to fifteen passes of the thumb walking technique to the area of interest. Do you see a change in color or appearance?

Drawing Inferences from Stress Cues of the Foot

Now that you've practiced observing stress cues, it's time to draw inferences from them. The stress cue is the basic building block in constructing an image of the individual's stress pattern. The absence of a stress cue, the presence of a stress cue, and the characteristics of the stress cues are used to create an objective assessment of the individual's stress pattern and overall health. An image of the foot's stress pattern thus forms the basis of client evaluation and helps you determine a plan of action. (See "S. O. A. P. P. Formula.")

Stress cue characteristics: magnitude, location, client opinion

The characteristics of the stress cue provide you with a means of measuring stress. The magnitude of the stress cue, its location, and the level of the client's stress awareness all provide information you can develop into a plan of action. Included in the plan are how many sessions will be required to achieve results.

In making an assessment, you reach conclusions about the impact of stress on the foot, the reflex area, and the body. Three basic techniques measure stress response: (1) The Foot Stress Scale describes the range along which stress adaptation takes place on the

Press and Assess Stress Cues

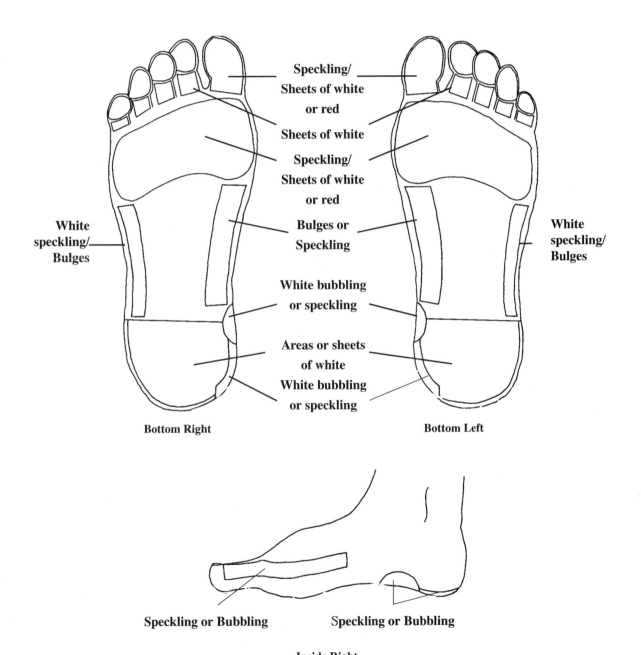

Speckling/
Sheets of white
or red

Sheets of white

Speckling/
Sheets of white
or red

Bulges or
Speckling

White bubbling
or speckling

Areas or sheets
of white

White bubbling
or speckling

White
speckling/
Bulges

White
speckling/
Bulges

Bottom Right

Bottom Left

Speckling or Bubbling

Speckling or Bubbling

Inside Right

foot, (2) The Reflex Stress Scale describes the range of stress adaptation reflected in the foot's reflexes, (3) The Body Stress Scale provides an opportunity for the reflexologist to compare his or her findings about stress adaptation to the individual's feelings about his or her stress level

Evaluating the Foot Stress Cue

The presence of a foot stress cue indicates an adaptation to stress. In evaluating foot stress cues, the reflexologist measures stress by considering the characteristics and magnitude of the stress cue. The measurement of the stress cue is seen as ranging from mild to moderate to extreme. The terms alarm, adaptation and exhaustions mirror this range and are utilized to evaluate the impact of stress. These terms parallel those of Selye and his stress theory.

In general, the more extreme the stress cue: (1) The more deeply ingrained the pattern of stress, (2) The greater the potential for the individual's awareness of stress and stress-related health problems, and (3) The more sessions and conditioning by pressure technique application will be required to achieve results and change the pattern of stress.

The Foot Stress Scale charts measurements of the commonly observed stress cues. For example, curled toes are noted to range from an alarm level of stress adaptation (single toe) to adaptive (several toes) to exhausted (extreme curl). Just as Selye saw age in terms of alarm (young person), adaptation (middle aged person) and exhaustion (older person), you will notice that stress cue measurements frequently parallel the age of the individual.

Alarm stage

In the *alarm stage of adaptation*, the stress cue shows signs of a lesser stress that has been adapted to over a shorter period of time or a stress that has little impact. If the stress is a recent event, the body is in the process of learning how to cope, and a lesser amount of technique application will be required to cause a change in stress level. Immediate change is possible because the stress pattern is not deeply ingrained, and merely interrupting the stress can reshape and condition the stress pattern.

In the *alarm stage of adaptation,* the foot may be sensitive to very sensitive to untouchable in response to pressure technique application. The foot thus shows signs of an immediate stress being adapted to by the body right now. Examples include illness, accident or stress. It can be (1) a short-term stress of such magnitude as to register ponderable disturbance or (2) a long-term, chronic stress that is currently active and acute.

In the *adaptive stage*, the stress cue shows signs of a stress adapted to over a period of time that has created some impact. The stress has been ingrained as a learning experience.

Adaptive stage

It is also possible that a recent stress of some magnitude has caused the body to adapt to considerable stress quickly. Examples include illness, accident or stress. In any case, consistency of technique application over time will be required to cause a change in stress level. Some immediate change may be possible as technique application interrupts stress sufficiently to cause a shift in the stage of adaptation.

In the *exhaustion stage of adaptation*, the stress cue shows signs of a stress adapted to over a lengthy time period. The stress has been deeply ingrained as a learning experience. OR: A recent stress of considerable magnitude has occurred, such as a serious accident, injury, illness, or emotional stress. Either will require regular technique application over a length of time to produce long-term results. Immediate change is possible as technique application interrupts current stress. A shift in stage of adaptation is possible over time.

Exhaustion stage

Drawing Foot Stress Inferences

In making foot stress inferences, the reflexologist considers the characteristics of the stress cue. Not only is a stress cue described as, for example, puffy, but the quality of puffiness is also measured and graded. The net result is accurate rating of the stage of adaptation. In addition, further inferences about stress patterns can be drawn.

To practice making inferences, once again (1) Consider the photographs, (2) Consider each stress cue, and (3) See if you can match it to a description of a stage of adaptation on the Foot Stress Scale. The left-hand column lists the stress cues. The other columns list the three stages of adaptation with stress cue characteristics listed under each. Select the stress cue and then find the column that best describes the characteristics you have found in that stress cue.

Drawing Foot Stress Inferences

• Note the stress cues on each foot.
• Once you have identified the stress cues, consider the level of adaptation of each stress cue and each foot as a whole.
• Now, compare and contrast the cues and inferences among all three.

See p. 232 for Author's Assessment.

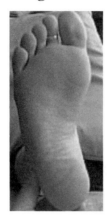
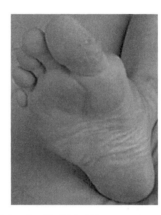
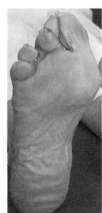

Once you have assessed each stress cue individually, consider the overall pattern of adaptation. Are most of the stress cues listed in the same column; thus, in the same stage of adaptation? Or are they of varied stages of adaptation? Are many of the stress cues gathered in one part of the foot, such as in the toes? Do the various parts of the foot differ in stages of adaptation?

These further inferences provide more depth to your evaluation. A stress cue that shows an adaptive level of other stress cues may be an indicator of an isolated stress incident, such as an accident or a foot injury. Stress cues that share adaptive level throughout only one part of the foot, such as the toes, are an indicator of a particular pattern of stress. Stress cues of similar levels throughout the foot show the overall level of stress adaptation.

Once again, consider the foot. What is your assessment of the overall pattern of adaptation by the foot? Is it the same as the level of adaptation by the other foot?

Evaluating the Reflex Areas Stress Pattern

Next, you'll be using the foot stress cue observations and inferences to identify the type of stress pattern. You'll be matching stress cues with reflex areas.

How stressed is a particular reflexive area or part of the foot? Now that you have observed the foot stress cues, it's time to consider whether or not a reflex area(s) of the foot is under stress. Once

Foot Stress Scale

Stress Cue	Level of Stress Adaptation		
	Alarm	**Adaptation**	**Exhaustion**
Visual Stress Cues			
Texture	Puffiness	Thickness, callousing	Callousing, extreme puffiness, entire foot puffy
Color	Some white speckling	White speckling	Whole foot very white, red, or blue
Foot Feature	Bunion, slight	Angled	Extreme angle, red
	Bulge/bump, puffy	Puffy to thick	Very puffy or thick
	Corn	Reddened, painful	Clear, painful
	Curled or crooked toe	Several toes	Most toes, knobby joints, extreme curl
	Low arch	Lower than most	No arch
	Lined arch	Lined arch with epi-center	Ingrained, lined arch with epi-center
	High arch	Higher than most	Extremely high
	Longer second toe	Much longer than other toes	Much longer and curled second toe with calloused tip
	Tailor's bunion	Calloused	Calloused, angled
	Toenail	Thick	Very thick
	Wear spot, 1 or 2 toes	Three toes	All toes
Touch Stress Cues	Puffiness	Thickness	Hard tonus, callousing
Sensitivity Stress Cues	Sharp, little tone	Sharp, deep	Aching, wide area
Press & Assess Stress Cues	White speckling	Streaks of red/white, white bumps	Raised white bumps, sheets of red/white

again, your observations and inferences about foot stress cues are noted when talking to a client or writing a report about the client. This provides objective information on which to base your evaluation and inferences about the reflex stress cue and pattern.

The location and patterns of the stress cue are the basic building blocks to construct an image of reflexive stress patterns. Again, the characteristic and magnitude of the stress cue provides certain predictable features. Size matters. The location of a stress cue is assessed according to the reflex area chart. The chart is a map of the body's plan for adaptation to stress as it relates to body parts. The reflex chart tells you where to look for stress cues and patterns of stress cues.

Evaluating the Reflex Stress Cue

How do you know when adaptation to stress by the reflex or reflexes has taken place? Counting stress cues, noting location, and assessing the adaptive level of each provides a picture of the reflex stress pattern. Can you pinpoint a reflex area associated with the foot stress cue? Is there a part of the foot such as the toes associated with several stress cues? Is there a pattern of stress cues associated with, for example, the skeletal system?

Is there a small concentrated area of stress impact, such as a reflex area reflecting two or more stress cues OR a reflex reflecting one or more exhausted or extremely sensitive stress cues.

Drawing Reflex Stress Inferences

• Note the stress cues and draw foot stress inferences for each foot.
• Referring to the Reflex Stress Scale, make reflex stress cue observations and inferences for each foot.
• Compare and contrast the feet.
See p. 108 for Author's Assessment.

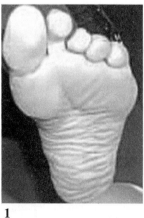 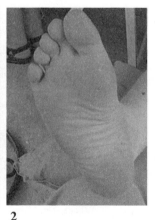 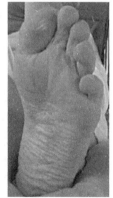

1   2   3

Reflex Stress Scale

Consider the foot stress cues. Consider the type of stress cue, such as alarm, and the location of each. Consider the type, number, and location of the stress cues to create a picture of the pattern of stress This information will give you an objective view of the individual's stress pattern.

Location of Stress Cue	Reflex Area Stress Cue Observation			Reflex Area Stress Cue Inferences
Part of Foot	Number of Alarm Stress Cues	Number of Adapted Stress Cues	Number of Exhausted Stress Cues	Reflex Areas
Toes	3 or more	2 or more	1 or more	Head, brain, sinus, jaw, teeth, neck, throat, thyroid, parathyroid
Base of toes	3 or more	2 or more	1 or more	Eye/Ear, Tops of shoulders
Ball of foot	3 or more	2 or more	1 or more	Upper back, lung / chest, heart, shoulder
Arch	3 or more	2 or more	1 or more	Stomach, Liver/ gallbladder, pancreas, adrenal glands, arm elbow, kidneys, colon, small intestines, back
Heel	3 or more	2 or more	1 or more	Colon, reproductive organs, lower back, tailbone
Inside of foot	3 or more	2 or more	1 or more	Back, uterus/prostate
Outside of foot	3 or more	2 or more	1 or more	Arm, elbow, hip, knee, ovary/testicle
Top of foot	3 or more	2 or more	1 or more	Head, neck, upper back

Next consider if there is a concentration of stress cues throughout a part of the foot such as the toes, for example, three or more alarm stress cues, two or more adapted stress cues, one or more exhausted stress cues in the toes.

Stress cues throughout every part of the foot indicate a generalized pattern of reflex stress. A generalized pattern is reflected by two or more regions in any one foot showing adaptation, such as the toes and the ball of the foot; one or more regions showing exhaustion; two or more extremely sensitive regions; a majority of the glands or organs within a system showing stress cues, such as three of the five endocrine glands or three or more stressed reflex areas within a zone.

Drawing Reflex Stress Inferences

The Reflex Stress Scale has been developed to provide a basic technique of reflex stress assessment. The left-hand column lists the possible location of stress cues. The right-hand columns list the number of stress cues and the stage of adaptation of the stress cues.

A reflex stress inference is made by considering the pattern of stress cues. The location, type (stage of adaptation), and number of stress cues combine together to indicate the pattern of stress. A reflexive stress pattern is established if a sufficient number of stress cues of a particular magnitude is present.

To practice this technique, consider the stress cues on a foot. (1) Count the exhausted stress cues, the adapted stress cues, and the alarm stress cues. (2) Consider the location of each stress cue. (3) Tally up the type, number, and location of stress cues. (4) Create a reference chart similar to the one shown as the Reflex Stress Scale.

Evaluating the Body Stress Pattern

Now that you have objectified your findings, it's time to compare those results with the individuals' response to stress. How stressed is this individual and how aware is he or she of his or her stress level? Perception of stress helps measure it. The reflexologist focuses on such questions about body stress by (1) listening to the individual or (2) asking questions of the individual. Both methods help the reflexologist confirm, refute, or change his or her assessment of the impact of stress on the individual. These responses and

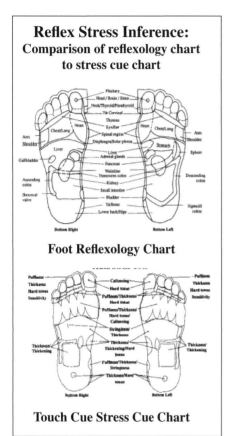

Reflex Stress Inference:
Comparison of reflexology chart
to stress cue chart

Foot Reflexology Chart

Touch Cue Stress Cue Chart

general comments are measured against your own findings. In addition, the client who hears a question that speaks to his or her health problem with the demonstrable sign of a stress cue will become convinced that you are a skilled practitioner of a valued service.

When do you ask a question? You ask a question when you encounter a stress cue or a stress cue pattern of such magnitude that it stands out among other stress cues and patterns. Consider asking a question when there are three alarm stress cues in a reflex area or region of the foot, two adapted stress cues, or one exhausted or very sensitive stress cue.

There are some rules of thumb in successful interviewing. First, the technique of interviewing an individual about his or her stress response takes practice. Secondly, the skill in asking the right number of questions. Asking too many questions will interrupt the relaxation provided by the session. It could also give the individual the false perception that you have found problems that he or she should worry about. Ask a minimal amount of questions to be successful in gauging the impact of stress on the individual. After all your goal is to determine a stage of adaptation for your observations. You have drawn your inferences, now it's time to see if they agree with the individual's perceptions of his or her body and health situation.

Ask questions of a broad, general nature. A question that is phrased, "Does your neck bother you?" is of a broad, general nature. It allows the individual to respond in a variety of ways: How long the stress has been present; what impact they're feeling, if any; and whether they consider it a problem. Ask follow-up question such as, "How long has it bothered you?" or "Do you consider it a problem?"

Evaluating Body Stress Cues

Once you have asked questions about the individual's stress pattern, it is time to evaluate compare and contrast your findings with the individual's responses. There are two basic responses to a question such as "Does your neck bother you?" – yes and no, however, there are shades of meaning. The skilled reflexologist reads between the lines. Below are responses with an interpretation of their real meaning.

"Yes." tells you that the individual is feeling the impact of stress and further questions or comments will fill in the picture.

"Yes, right now." The individual is reporting that he or she is bothered by a stress-related condition currently.

"Yes, once in a while." The individual is reporting that he or she feels the effects of a stress occasionally. This indicates a stress pattern of less wear and tear that has not been deeply ingrained. Keep in mind, however, that the individual may not be accurately reporting his or her stress adaptation. It may be deeply ingrained but overridden by the individual.

"Yes, it comes and goes." The individual is reporting that the stress recurs on a regular basis. It is ingrained to the point that the wear-and-tear pattern is becoming conditioned as a stress response. The individual's ability to rebound from a stress event such as an illness takes place within limits.

"Yes, all the time." The individual is reporting that he or she feels the effects of chronic stress. The wear-and-tear pattern of stress has ingrained itself over a lengthy time period. If the individual names a disorder or reports a diagnosis, the stress response has been present long enough to acquire a name such as "my neck problem" or "The doctors tell me I have scoliosis." Also, a report of a stress event such as a car accident, operation, illness, or emotional distress is a clue to possible extensive wear and tear.

"No." can have several meanings and can tell you something about the individual's perception of stress and his or her ability to cope with it.

"No, it doesn't bother me." By giving a negative response to a single question about a stress cue on the foot, the individual, thus, is reporting that impact of the stress is negligible and he or she has the ability to cope with the stress.

"No, it did bother me." By giving this response, the individual is reporting that he or she is not aware of the stress at this time and has learned to adapt and cope with the stress.

"No, nothing really bothers me." By giving a negative response to almost every question, this individual may be unaware of the effects of stress altogether. The individual has learned to cope by overriding his or her stress mechanism. Continuous overstressing can lead to exhaustion.

Drawing Body Stress Inferences

To draw body stress inferences, the reflexologist categorizes the individual's perceptions. For example, a question such as "Does your back bother you?" is asked to test your theory about the individual's level of stress adaptation in reference to their back. See the "Body Stress Scale, pp 92- 93.

To practice making body stress inferences, note "Drawing Body Stress Inferences" below. In addition, try this exercise. Refer to the following pages and start at the toes of the individual's foot. Consider whether or not there is any stress cue or pattern of stress cues that has drawn your attention. Note the number or letter of the alphabet in the illustration which indicates the location of a stress cue or cues. Note the question related to the number or letter of the alphabet. Consider the appropriateness of asking a general or more specific question of the individual. Now, ask the question to clarify your assessment. Your goal is to determine whether or not the individual perceives as a problem the stress pattern that you have observed. Go on to each part of the foot.

Drawing Body Stress Inferences

• Consider the stress cues, foot stress inferences and reflex stress inferences.
• Referring to the following pages, which, if any, questions would be appropriate to ask of the owners of each foot?

See p. 108 for Author's Assessment.

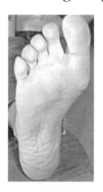
4

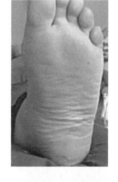
5

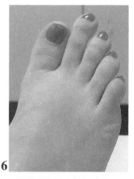
6

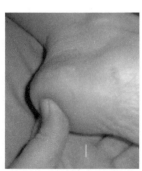
7

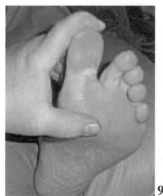
8

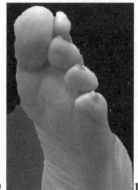
9

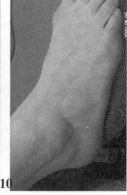
10

Body Stress Scale

Consider asking a question if any stress cue is of sufficient magnitude to draw your attention or if any pattern of stress cues draws your attention. This chart should serve only as a guide and not as a diagnostic tool.

Toes

A. Do you ever have headaches or problems with your upper back or neck?

1. Do you have headaches?

2. Do your sinuses bother you? Do you have sinus headaches?

3. Does your neck bother you? Does your throat bother you?

4. Does your jaw bother you?

5. Do you have teeth problems? Do you have gum problems?

6. Do you have memory problems?

6a. Do you have highs and lows of energy?

Base of Toes

B. Do your eyes and ears bother you?

7. Do your ears bother you? Do your eyes bother you?

8. When you get up quickly, do you occasionally get dizzy?

9. Do your eyes bother you?

10. Do you feel tension on the tops of your shoulders?

Ball of the Foot

C. Have you ever had problems in the back or chest region?

11. Do you feel tension in the upper back? Chest?

12. Do you feel tension between the shoulder blades?
In the chest? In the neck? Upper back? Do you wear
high heels regularly?

13. Do you feel tension between the shoulder blades?

14. Do you get heavy chest colds in the winter?

15. Does your shoulder bother you?

16. Are you under a lot of stress?

17. Do you get acid indigestion?

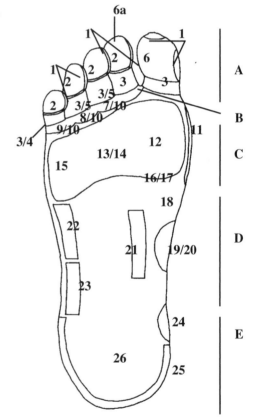

Arch of the Foot

D. Does your midback to lower back ever bother you?

18. Do you have allergies? Asthma? Hay fever? Sinus problems? Feelings of total exhaustion?

19. Do you experience sudden drops in energy? In the afternoon?

20. Does your stomach bother you?

21. Have you had problems with your kidneys?

22. Does your arm bother you?

23. Do you have digestive problems?

Heel

E. Does your lower back bother you?

24. Does your lower back bother you?

25. Have you injured your lower back?

26. Do you have digestive problems? Lower back problems?

Top of Foot

F. Does your chest or upper back bother you?

27. Do you get numbness in the fingers? Do your hands get cold?

28. Do you feel tension in the upper back or chest?

29. Do you get sudden drops of energy in the afternoon?

30. Have you had problems with your kidneys?

31. Do you have digestive problems?

32. Have you had reproductive problems?

Outside of Foot

G. Do your legs and hips ever bother you?

33. Does your knee, hip, leg or lower back bother you?

34. Does your hip bother you? Have you ever had sciatica?

Inside of Foot

H. Does your back bother you?

35. Does your neck bother you?

36. Do you feel tension between the shoulder blades?

37. Does your back bother you, particularly in the middle?

38. Does your lower back bother you?

39. Have you ever injured your lower back or tailbone?

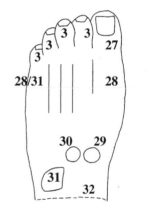

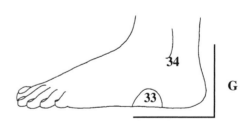

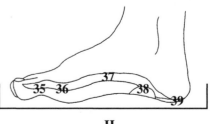

93

Assessing the Foot Session Pattern

Now that you've learned how to identify stress cues, draw inferences from them and evaluate them, it's time to practice putting all skills together to make an integrated assessment session. Once again, assessing the foot is a skill acquired by the reflexologist to identify areas of the foot for technique application emphasis. The information you gather serves as a gauge for how much technique to apply, a reference point to measure how much change has taken place, and an indicator of meeting the individual's goals. (See "The Session.")

Assessing the foot allows the reflexologist to reach some conclusions about the individual's response to stress. Two qualities of stress response are noted: (1) the level of adaptation, such as alarm, adaptation, or exhaustion, and (2) the type of response, such as foot stress, reflex stress, or body stress. Thus, the foot, the reflex, and the body can be evaluated for stress.

The following session pattern provides you with an opportunity to practice observing and evaluating the foot in a systematic manner. Each segment is organized with visual stress cue observations first, then touch / sensitivity, followed by press and assess stress cue observations. A summary of observations and an evaluation of foot, reflex, and body stress inferences completes the segment. The goal of the completed session pattern is to create an assessment of the individual's pattern of stress. This session pattern should serve only as a guide and not a diagnostic tool.

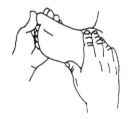

Observe the foot as you look it over for cuts, callouses, and bruises. What is you general impression of the foot? Is it a thick foot? A thin foot? An average foot? What do you consider the most outstanding visual cue on the foot? Are there several significant cues? Do the visual cues center around one part of the foot, such as the ball of the foot? How does this foot compare in general to the feet of individuals of the same gender and age group? Does the foot show what you might expect with respect to stress cues?

The Toes

head / brain / sinus

pituitary / hypothalamus

jaw / teeth / gums

thyroid / parathyroid

neck / throat / seventh cervical

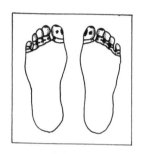

1 Look at the toes. Observe the visual cues. Are the toes straight? Crooked? How crooked? Curled? How curled? Which toes? Do the toes stand independently from each other? Are there wear spots on the toes? Which toes? Is there callousing? Where? How much? What color? On both feet? Are the toes puffy? The ball of the toe? The stem? Which toe(s)? Are any of the toenails thickened? Are there any corns?

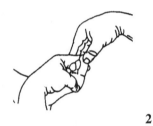

1

2 Apply the thumb walking technique to the toes. Consider the touch cues. Is the ball of the toe sensitive to pressure? Light pressure? What do you feel? Puffiness? Thickness? Hard tonus? Where? If there are wear spots, do they feel markedly different in tonus from the surrounding area?

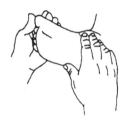

2

3 Apply the thumb walking technique to walk up the toes. What do you feel? Is the stem of the toe sensitive to pressure? Do you feel puffiness? Thickness? Hard tonus? Where?

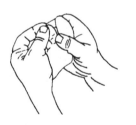

4 Apply the hook and back up technique to the pituitary / hypothalamus reflex area. Is it sensitive? How sensitive? What do you feel?

5 Roll the tip of the finger over the tip of the big toe. Is it sensitive? What do you feel?

3

6 Apply the finger walking technique to the seventh cervical reflex area around the base of the big toe. Is there sensitivity? Do you feel hard tonus?

7 Apply the thumb walking technique to the thyroid / parathyroid / neck / throat reflex area, the stem of the big toe. Is there sensitivity? What do you feel? Puffiness? Thickness? Stringiness? Thumb walk across the area from the opposite direction. What do you feel?

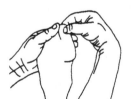

4

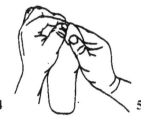

5

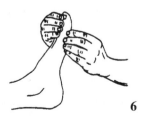

6

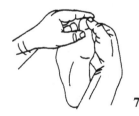

7

95

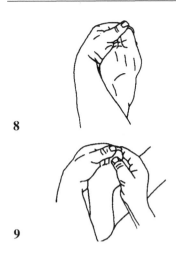

8 Hold the toe back in a stretched position to make a press and assess observation of it. Do sheets of white coloration appear?

9 Press the toe with the flat of your thumb for several seconds. Lift your thumb. Do you see bubbling or speckling?

Consider the overall picture you have observed in the toes. Have you noted multiple stress cues? In the big toe? In all the small toes? Were the observed stress cues also sensitive to pressure technique application? Do you consider the toes to show signs of alarm, adaptation, or exhaustion? Do you consider the stress cues to be local, regional, or general in nature? Are there a sufficient number of stress cues to prompt you to ask the individual about his or her perception of stress in a corresponding body part? Note the overall stress pattern and keep it in mind as you work through the foot. Compare the stress pattern in the toes to that of the base of the toes.

Base of the Toes

eye / ear

tops of shoulders

10 Observe the base of the toes. Are there visible wear spots? Where? Can you see the base of the toes or is it concealed by puffiness from the ball of the foot?

11 Apply the thumb walking technique to the eye / ear / tops of the shoulders reflex area.

11a Change your working hand and walk from the opposite direction.

Consider the touch stress cues. Is there sensitivity? Where? Between the second and third toes? The third and fourth? The fourth and fifth? What does it feel like to you? An irregular surface? Puffiness? Thickening sheets of tonus? Thickened tonus? Hard tonus? Is there an overall pattern of stress or one that is localized to an area or areas? Compare the stress cues you have observed in the base of the toes to those you observed in the toes. Are there multiple stress cues in both? Are both uniform in stress cue observations and stress inferences?

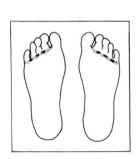

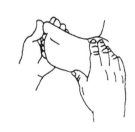

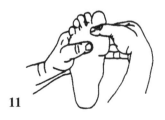

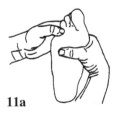

Ball of the Foot

chest / lung / heart / breast

solar plexus / diaphragm

shoulder

upper back / between the shoulders

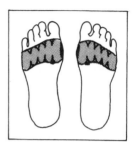

12 Observe the ball of the foot for visual stress cues. What is your overall impression? Is there callousing? Where? How thick? Over how large an area? How thick is it? What color, if any? Is there a bunion? How extreme is it? Is it red and swollen? Is there a tailor's bunion? How calloused is it?

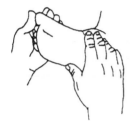
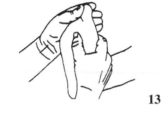

12   **13**

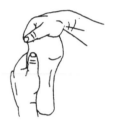

14

13 Apply the thumb walking technique to the ball of the foot. What touch cues do you note? Is there sensitivity? Where? What do you feel? Is there thickening? Thickness? Hard tonus? Stringiness? Puffiness? Where? Over how large an area?

14 Apply the thumb walking technique to the shoulder area. Is there sensitivity? Thickness? Hard tonus? Apply the thumb walking technique to the solar plexus/diaphragm area. Is it sensitive to pressure? Light pressure? Moderate pressure? What do you feel? A stringy or thickened band? General thickness?

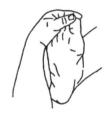

15

15 Hold the foot back and make a press and assess observation of it. Do sheets of white or red, white speckling, or white bubbling appear? Where? Is there visible pulsing from white to red in the solar plexus reflex area?

16 Press the ball of the foot with the flat of the thumb in the area of interest. Lift the thumb. Does speckled or bubbled white coloration appear?

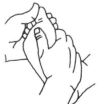

16

Consider the stress cues you have observed in the foot thus far. Are there multiple stress cues in each of the toes, the base of the toes, and the ball of the foot? Is there an overall pattern of stress or a localized one? What reflex area observations have you made?

Arch of the Foot (Above the Waistline)

Right Foot / Left Foot

adrenal gland / adrenal gland

liver/gallbladder / spleen

stomach (part) / stomach

pancreas (part) / pancreas

kidney (top of) / kidney (top of)

midback/spine / midback / spine

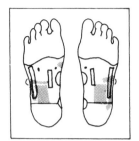

17 Observe the arch of the foot for visual stress cues. Is it a high arch? A low arch? Is there thickness? Callousing? Puffiness? Where?

18 Apply the thumb walking technique to the foot. Establish the boundaries for the area – the waistline, tendon, and solar plexus reflex area – to map touch stress cues. What do you feel? Thickness? Hard tonus? Stringiness? Where? Over how large an area? Is there a shape to the observed tonus?

19 Apply the thumb walking technique from another direction. Does your picture of what you feel

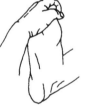

17

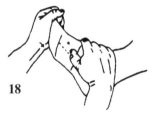

18

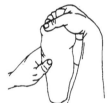

19

This area of the foot includes a long list of reflex areas with many possibilities for stress cues. Observing the touch stress cues takes practice. Use the above list of reflex areas as a checklist for the site of possible touch stress cues. Approach the site of each reflex area from several directions to fully consider the possibility of a touch stress cue.

Arch of the Foot (Below the Waistline)

Right Foot / Left Foot

colon / colon

ileocecal valve / sigmoid colon

small intestine / small intestine

kidney (part of) / kidney (part of)

lower back/hip/pelvis / lower back / hip / pelvis

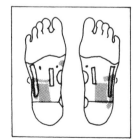

20 Observe the arch of the foot for visual cues. Note any callousing, puffiness, or thickness.

21 Apply thumb walking technique to the foot. Establish the boundaries of the area –the waistline, the tendon, and the heel – to map touch cues. What do you feel? Thickness? Hard tonus? Is there shape to what you feel?

22 Apply the thumb walking technique from another direction. Does your picture of what you feel change?

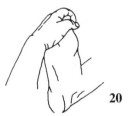 **20**
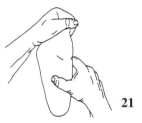 **21**
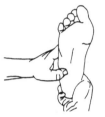 **22**

23 Observe the foot. Is there a bump at the base of the fifth metatarsal, midway on the outside of the foot?

24 (Right foot) Apply the hook and back up technique to the ileocecal area. Is there sensitivity?

25 (Left foot) Apply the hook and back up technique to the sigmoid colon area. Is there sensitivity? Do you feel hard tonus?

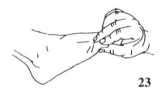 **23**
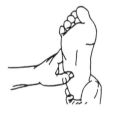 **24**
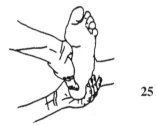 **25**

Consider the stress cues you have observed in the foot thus far. Are there multiple stress cues in any of the toes, the base of the toes, the ball of the foot, and the arch? Is there an overall pattern of stress, a regional one, or a localized one? What reflex area observations have you made?

Heel

lower back

pelvis

colon

26 Observe the heel for visual stress cues. Is there callousing? Where? Around the heel? Over the entire heel? How thick? Are there cracks or breaks in the skin?

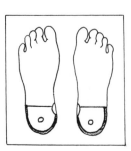

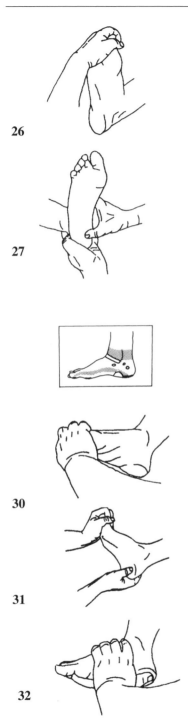

26

27

30

31

32

27 Apply the thumb walking technique to the heel. Is there sensitivity? Thickness? Hard tonus?

28 Position the foot. Apply direct pressure to the center of the heel with the flat of the thumb make a press and assess observation of it. Observe any change in coloration in the area surrounding the thumb.

29 Lift the thumb. Note color.

Once again, consider the stress cues you have observed on the foot thus far.

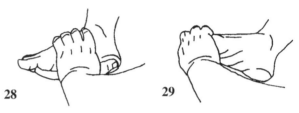

28   **29**

Inside of the Foot

spine

tailbone

bladder

rectum

uterus / prostate

30 Observe the foot for visual stress cues. Is there puffiness? Callousing? Where? The heel? Ball of foot? The big toe?

31 Apply the thumb walking technique to the tailbone reflex area. Is there sensitivity? What do you feel? Hard tonus? If the tailbone reflex area is markedly sensitive, make a press and assess observation of it. Position the flat of the thumb near the edge of the heel.

32 Apply direct pressure with the flat of the thumb and observe the area surrounding the thumb. Do white bubbles or white speckles appear? Where? How much? Can you feel the bubbling when you run your fingers over the area? Lift your thumb. Does the previously observed coloration remain?

33 Apply the thumb walking technique to the bladder / lower back reflex area. Is there sensitivity to pressure? Light pressure? How does it feel to your touch? Puffy? Thick? Hard? Stringy band embedded in the tonus?

34 Apply the thumb walking technique to the spinal reflex area. Establish the boundaries for the reflex areas; waistline for midback, ball of foot for between the shoulder blades, and big toe for the neck. Is there sensitivity? Where? What do you feel? Puffiness? Thickness? Hard tonus? If the area is markedly sensitive or draws your attention through visual and touch cues, make a press and assess observation of it.

35 Stretch the skin taut. Is there any change in the coloration of the area? Any bubbling? White speckling?

36 Observe the inside of the ankle for visual stress cues. Do you notice general puffiness? A specific area of puffiness in the uterus/ prostate area?

37 Apply the rotating on a point technique to the area. Is there sensitivity? Do you feel hard tonus?

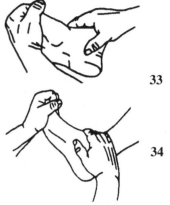

Consider the stress cues you have observed in the foot thus far. Have you observed an overall consistency to the stress cues?

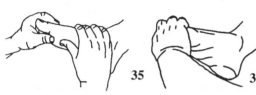

Outside of the Foot

arm

hip / sciatic

knee / leg

ovary / testicle

lower back / pelvis

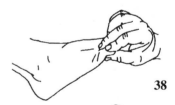

38 Observe the outside of the foot for visual stress cues. Is there puffiness? Thickness? A bump?

39 Apply the thumb walking technique to the arm reflex area. What do you feel? Thickness? Hard tonus?

40 Apply the finger walking technique to the hip / sciatic reflex area. Is there sensitivity?

41 Apply the thumb walking technique to the knee / leg reflex area. Is there sensitivity? What do you feel? Thickness? Hard tonus?

42 Apply the thumb walking technique to the ovary / testicle reflex area. Is there sensitivity? Hard tonus?

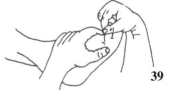

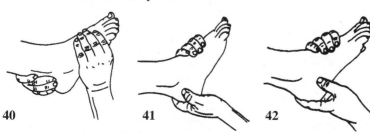

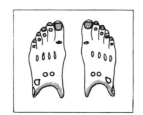

Top of the Foot

head

neck

tops of shoulders

chest / breast

lung / shoulder

upper back

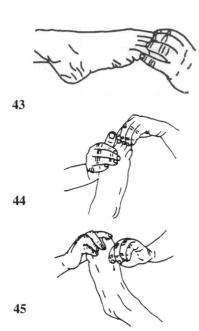

43

44

45

43 Observe the top of the foot for visual stress cues. Note corns, toenails, tendons that stand out, bumps, bulges, puffiness.

44 Apply the finger walking technique to the tops of the toes. Is there sensitivity? What do you feel? Thickness? Hard tonus especially around the joints?

45 Apply the finger walking technique to the foot. Is there sensitivity? Hard tonus? Stringiness? Where?

46 Apply the multiple finger walking technique to the foot. Is there sensitivity? Thickness? Bumps of hard tonus? Is bulge puffy to the touch? Thick? Hard?

47 Apply the thumb walking technique to the lymphatic / groin / fallopian tube reflex area. Do you feel puffiness? Hard, thickened tonus?

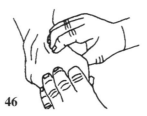

46

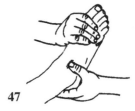

47

Summary

Consider the overall picture you have observed in the foot. Are the visual, touch, press and assess, and sensitivity cues about equal throughout the foot? Or do you note local, concentrated areas of stress cues? Have you observed a region of the foot, such as the toes, that shows more stress cues than the others? Is there a general pattern of stress cues throughout the foot? Do you note a general lack of stress cues?

As you work through the second foot, compare it to the first foot. Are the two feet about equal in stress cues? Does one show markedly more stress cues than the other?

Assessment Summary Chart

To assess the foot (1) Select a part of the foot, such as the toes, for assessment. (2) Review the reflex areas in that part of the foot. (3) Determine whether or not there are any foot stress cues associated with the reflex area. (4) Consider the comments made by the individual about his or her response to stress. This chart should be used only as a guide and not as a diagnostic tool.

Assessment Summary Chart			
Foot Part	**Foot Stress Cue**	**Reflex Stress Inference**	**Body Stress Response**
Ball of toes	Puffiness, thickness, hard tonus	Head / brain / sinus	Headaches, sinus problems
	Callousing	Head	Headaches
	Wear spots		Headaches, neck/upper back tension, facial pain, teeth/gum/jaw problems, hearing problems
	Puffiness, sensitivity	Sinus	Sinus problems, neck problems
	Thickness/hard tonus, sensitivity		Sinusitis, sinus headaches, neck problems
	Overlapping toes, bulge in big toe	Brain	Memory problems
	Longer second toe		Blood sugar level problems
Stem of toes	Sensitivity, thickness to hard tonus, crooked toes	Neck	Neck tension to neck problems
	Sensitivity, puffiness to thickness	Throat	Sore throat, sinus problems
	Sensitivity, thickened to stringy tonus	Thyroid / parathyroid	Low energy
	Thickness to hard tonus, wear spots	Teeth / gum / jaws	Jaw injury/problems, dental problems

Assessment Summary Chart			
Foot Part	**Foot Stress Cue**	**Reflex Stress Inference**	**Body Stress Response**
Base of toes	Thickening to thickened to hard tonus	Tops of shoulders	Tension in the tops of the shoulders, shoulder
	Sensitivity, thickening to thickened to hard tonus, wear spot	Eyes	Eye strain
	Thickened to hardened tonus, sensitivity, wear spots	Eyes	Eye problems
	Sensitivity, thickening tonus, wear spot	Ear	Ringing in the ears
	Hard tonus, wear spot, sensitivity	Ear	Hearing or ear problems
	Hard tonus, wear spot, sensitivity	Inner ear	Dizziness (such as when rising from a chair), vertigo, balance
Ball of foot	Visual puffiness, thickened to hard to stringy tonus, sensitivity	Solar plexus	General tension, emotional response, breathing
	Speckled coloring to sheets of white/red, thickened to hardened tonus	Lungs	Frequent colds, lung problems
	Thickened to hardened tonus, sensitivity, puffiness	Chest / breast	Tension in the chest, breast problems
	Puffiness to thickened to hardened tonus, white speckling on a red background to sheets of white, callousing	Heart	Tension in the chest, heart problems
	Thickening to thickened to hard tonus, callousing, tailor's bunion	Shoulder	Shoulder injury/problems

Assessment Summary Chart

Foot Part	Foot Stress Cue	Reflex Stress Inference	Body Stress Response
Ball of foot	Speckled coloring to sheets of white/red, thickened to hard tonus, callousing	Upper back	Upper back tension/problems, whiplash
	Callousing, thickened to hard tonus, sensitivity	Arm	Arm problems such as weakness or aching, elbow, shoulder, or neck problems
Arch of foot	Sensitivity, thickened to hard tonus	Adrenal glands	Infection, asthma, allergies, hay fever, sinus problems/headaches, low energy
	Puffy to thickened tonus, visual puffiness, sensitivity	Pancreas	Low energy, highs and lows of energy, emotional stress
	Stringy to thickened to hard tonus, sensitivity	Gallbladder	Digestive problems, flatulence
	Callousing or visual puffiness, sensitivity, puffy to thickened to hard tonus	Kidney	Kidney problems, mid to lower back problems
	Stringy to thickened to hard tonus, sensitivity	Spleen	Anemia, immune response problems
	Visual puffiness/thickening, thickened to hard tonus, sensitivity	Stomach	Stomach problems, tension in the stomach
	Thickening to hard tonus	Small intestine	Digestive problems
	Callousing, thickening to hard tonus, sensitivity	Large intestine	Digestive problems, foot/knee/hip joint problems
	Thickened to hard tonus, sensitivity	Liver	Digestive problems, immune response problems

105

Assessment Summary Chart

Foot Part	Foot Stress Cue	Reflex Stress Inference	Body Stress Response
	Lines	Back	Spinal reflex area at the origin of lines indicates level of back tension
Heel	Callousing/cracking, thickened to hard tonus, sensitivity	Colon, lower back, hip, pelvis, reproductive organs	Digestive problems, lower back problems, reproductive problems
	Speckling/white bumps, sensitivity, hard tonus	Tailbone	Injury, lower back tension/ problems, digestive problems
	Puffiness, sensitivity, thickened to hard tonus	Rectum	Digestive problems, hemorrhoids
Inside of foot	Sensitivity, puffy to thickened to hard tonus, bump, visible speckling or other color	Spine	Injury, back tension/problems, digestive problems, reproductive problems
	Puffiness, sensitivity, redness, thickened to hard tonus	Bladder / lower back	Bladder problems, lower back problems
	Visual puffiness, sensitivity, thickened to hard tonus	Uterus / prostate	Reproductive problems
	Visual puffiness, thickened tonus	Sacroiliac	Lower back problems
Outside of foot	Sensitivity, puffy to thickened to hard tonus	Lower back, hip/ sciatic	Lower back tension/problems, sciatic problems

Assessment Summary Chart

Foot Part	Foot Stress Cue	Reflex Stress Inference	Body Stress Response
	Sensitivity, puffiness to thickened tonus	Knee / leg	Knee/leg problems
	Thickened to hard tonus	Elbow, knee	Digestive problems, elbow or knee problems
Top of foot (toes)	Thickened toenail, thickened to hard tonus, sensitivity, crooked or curled toes	Head/brain/sinus	Stress problems
	Corn	Neck	Headaches, neck aches or problems, shoulder problems
Top of foot (body of foot)	Taut tendons	Upper back	Upper back tension, whiplash
	Bulge, visual puffiness, thickened to hard tonus	Small intestine, large intestine	Digestive problems, shoulder problems
	Bump, hard tonus	Kidney	Kidney or urinary problems
	Bump, hard tonus	Pancreas	Low energy, highs and lows of energy
Ankle	Visual puffiness/thickness, puffy to thickened tonus, hard tonus	Lymphatic glands, fallopian tubes, groin, lower back	Ankle injury/swelling, reproductive problems, foot problems, lower back problems, foot problems

107

Author's Assessment

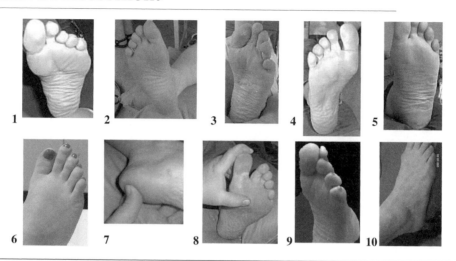

p. 86

1 Foot Stress Cues / Inferences: Bunion, several toes curled and pressing; wear spots, high and lined arch; callousing on the big toe, tailor's bunion / Adaptation stage
Reflex Stress Inferences: Ear, between the shoulder blades, upper back
Body Stress Inferences: Do you have hearing problems? Does your upper back bother you?
2 Foot Stress Cues / Inferences: High arch, lines, radiating from an epi-center, pressed toes, callousing on big toe / Adaptation stage
Reflex Stress Inferences: Mid-back, upper back, shoulders
Body Stress Inferences: Does your back bother you - mid to lower back?
3 Foot Stress Cues / Inferences: Longer second toe, skin texture in center of big toe, several curled toes, wear spots, toes pressed together, bunion, texture of arch surface / Exhaustion stage
Reflex Stress Inferences: Endocrine glands, mid back, ears
Body Stress Inferences: Do you get tired? Does your back bother you? How is your hearing?

p. 91

4 Foot Stress Cues / Inferences: Toes pressed together, calloused big toe, thickness in arch / Adaptation stage
Reflex Stress Inferences: Neck, shoulders, upper back, sinuses
Body Stress Inferences: Does your upper back bother you? Do your sinuses bother you?
5 Foot Stress Cues / Inferences: flat foot, lined arch, several curled toes, wear spots, toes pressed together / Adaptation stage

Reflex Stress Inferences: Digestive system, back
Body Stress Inferences: Does your digestion bother you? Your back?
6 Foot Stress Cues / Inferences: Much longer second toe / Adaptation stage
Reflex Stress Inferences: Head, neck, pancreas
Body Stress Inferences: Do you have neck problems? Headaches? Do you have highs and lows of energy?
7 Foot Stress Cues / Inferences: White raised bumps (press and assess stress cue), puffiness where heel meets foot / Adaptation stage
Reflex Stress Inferences: Tailbone, lower back
Body Stress Inferences: Does your tailbone or lower back bother you?
8 Foot Stress Cues / Inferences: White sheet in stem of big toe / Alarm stage
Reflex Stress Inferences: Throat, upper bronchial
Body Stress Inferences: Does your throat bother you?
9 Foot Stress Cues / Inferences: Extreme position of second toe; thickened toe nail; several toes pressing and curled / Exhaustion stage
Reflex Stress Inference: Head, neck
Body Stress Inference: Do you have memory problems?
10 Foot Stress Inferences: Localized puffy ankle; mottled color of whole foot, bunion, toes pressed together / Exhaustion stage
Reflex Stress Inferences: Hip, lower back
Body Stress Inferences: Does your hip bother you? Your back? *See also p. 232.*

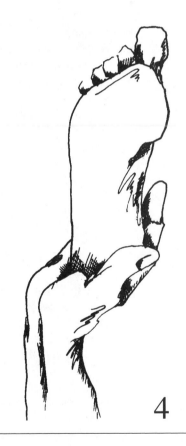

4

The Session

The Session

Putting the techniques together into a coherent pattern is in itself an important part of reflexology. You have learned patterns for applying technique, assessing stress cues, and considering the individual. The goal of the session is to combine these elements into an organized, consistent approach to get results, to create a relaxing experience, to relate your work in a credible manner and to document it for medical personnel or insurance claims.

The session pattern is a systematic, repeatable method of applying technique to the foot. Technique is applied to the entire foot at least once to contribute to the goal of relaxing the entire body and its stress mechanism. In addition, it affords you an opportunity to assess the foot in a systematic manner. Technique specifically tailored to the individual is then applied. The session includes: (1) working through a foot once to apply pressure technique to the entire foot and to observe stress cues on the entire foot and (2) working through the foot a second time, applying pressure technique to areas of emphasis (stress cues) selected during the first work through.

Going through the foot from top to bottom is a way of organizing a plan of action. It gives you an opportunity to gather your thoughts about the stress patterns, to create priorities for further technique application, and to seek information from the individual that clarifies their stress pattern.

Going through the foot a second time allows you to emphasize technique application appropriate to the individual's stress pattern. The individual's stress pattern may consist of a foot stress pattern, a reflex stress pattern, a body stress pattern, or any combination of the three. You want to match your technique application to the individual's stress pattern to produce optimal results. The skill you develop is the ability to customize your technique application to that individual.

The science of reflexology may be the application of pressure technique, but the art of reflexology is in your response to the individual as a whole. It is the final polish for the truly successful reflexologist. Each individual comes to you with a preset level of stress adaptation and predetermined goals for a session. Effectively and efficiently creating a relaxation response involves consideration of technique application during a session and over a series of sessions. The integrated foot reflexology session causes a relaxation response because it provides an appropriate level of pressure technique application. The goal of this chapter is to describe to you aspects of successful session planning.

The five-stage process described in this chapter is designed to guide you through the elements of a session. Providing a session is the application of technique appropriate to relax the stresses of a particular individual.

The goal of the session is to (1) Apply technique to the feet with a strategy appropriate to the stress cue observations and inferences; (2) Interview the individual to gather information about his or her stress history, relaxation goals, and expectations; (3) Develop a session strategy that best provides relaxation for that individual; (4) Plan a series of sessions; and (5) Document your work for medical personnel or insurance claims.

Applying Technique to the Foot

Once you've observed the stress cues and drawn inferences from them, it's time to apply technique to the feet with an appropriate strategy. Pressure technique strategy consists of how much pressure, how many passes, where and over how many sessions technique is applied. Every pair of feet is a puzzle with the question, "How can this foot best be unlocked from its pattern of stress?"

Philosophy of Technique Application to Relax Stress

Stress researcher Hans Selye noted the stereotypical response of the body to stress as a progression through the stages of adaptation: alarm, adaptation, and exhaustion. The reflexologist assesses the foot and notes the stages of adaptation. The reflexologist then elicits a relaxation response by applying a consistent program of pressure to the feet. The technique that is just right lulls the foot and body into a sense of relaxation. The right level of pressure unlocks tissues, relaxes muscles, and causes change. The goal is to balance technique application with the foot's state of stress adaptation: alarm, adaptation, or exhaustion.

Researchers have noted the importance of technique application appropriate to the individual and situation. In a 1996 article, two Chinese authors stated that it is necessary to apply reflexology technique at a level of an "effective stimulating strength." They hypothesized that frequency, duration, and intensity of technique application are all factors in determining the success of reflexology work. For example. "For children and young women,

111

light force is used, while we may exert heavy pressure on male patients who have big feet, and less sensitive skin."[1]

It is possible for pressure technique application to be insufficient to interrupt the stress mechanism. Heavily adapted stressed areas of the foot tend to resist weak signals or light pressure. Heavily adapted areas also require a sophisticated approach to unlock the Rubik's cube of stress.

The signal of pressure itself is a stressor. It changes from being a good stressor to being a bad stressor when it is applied beyond the ability of the individual's stage of adaptation to cope with its application. For example, too much pressure applied to the already exhausted feet of an individual may cause further exhaustion. The art of reflexology is to remain under the person's range of tolerance, not above it.

Creating Change With Technique Application

The reflexologist applies pressure techniques to the feet for the purpose of interrupting the individual's stress pattern. This is accomplished by matching the appropriate technique application with the particular area of emphasis on the foot. The overall goal is a pattern of technique application to stressed areas on the foot that results in a change in overall stress patterns.

In applying technique to the foot, first consider the response of the foot to pressure technique. An initial application of technique interrupts the pattern of stress. Technique application over several sessions conditions the foot and creates a change in overall stress pattern. Ongoing work educates the foot to respond to stress in the best possible manner.

The stereotypical response of the body to such pressure application is a progression through the stages of interruption, conditioning, and education. The stimulus of pressure interrupts stress and evokes a response of relaxation. Pressure technique applied consistently over time creates a conditioned, reflexive response. Such technique application interferes with the stress pattern on a frequency basis sufficient to create change. Continued technique application is an educational exercise within brain-organ dynamics.

[1.] Jinqui, Feng and Chunmei, Fan, "A Concept of the Strength of Stimulation in Reflexology," *1996 China Symposium Report*, China Reflexology Association, Beijing,1996

Next, consider the individual's initial pattern of stress adaptation. The rate at which a change in stress patterns takes place varies according to the individual's initial stress pattern – whether it is alarm, adaptation, or exhaustion. **Remember the Basic Rule of Foot Stress / Relaxation: The more the adaptation to stress over the longer the period of time: (1) The more pronounced the stress cue. (2) The more deeply ingrained the pattern of stress. (3) The greater the potential for the individual's awareness of stress and/or stress-related problems. (4) The more conditioning by pressure technique application will be required over a longer period of time to change the pattern of stress.**

To change a pattern of stress from any one stage of adaptation to another requires consistent, systematic technique application, including where to apply technique, how much pressure to apply, how many passes to make, and how many sessions are suggested. Your goal with technique strategy is to achieve the maximum effect with a minimum of effort. The most effective application of technique provides an appropriate level of challenge.

Technique Strategy

How much pressure to use, how frequently to apply that pressure, where to apply pressure, and how many sessions will be required are questions asked by the reflexologist in determining a technique procedure that will most efficiently and effectively relax and condition the foot. Consider the application of pressure technique to be an opportunity to shape up and exercise the foot. Just as any exercise program provides guidelines for working with the body, the reflexologist utilizes a strategy of exercise procedures to appropriately condition the foot.

Consider the evaluation of the foot discussed in the previous chapter. The patterns of stress encountered on a foot are measured according to alarm, adaptation, and exhaustion stages. The technique strategy you use to elicit a relaxation response will be matched to the patterns of stress adaptation. Pressure is your working tool. The amount of pressure, the number of passes, and the number of sessions reflect the reflexologist's basic questions of how much pressure to apply, how long to apply it, and where to apply it.

How Much Pressure to Apply

The reflexologist works with a "variable speed" thumb walking technique, with the ability to provide a variety of pressure levels from light to medium to heavy to any number of gradations in between. Observe the foot.

Consider the cues that you see and feel. Work for change in the area of the foot to which you are applying technique. Work within the comfort zone of the individual. Practice applying a variety of pressure levels to an area of the foot and note the response of each.

Light pressure

Light pressure is a level of pressure that interrupts stress and does not challenge it. Stress cues of exhaustion and extreme sensitivity, the foot of an older person, or an infant's foot call for a light touch. In addition, light pressure is a "warm-up" level of pressure for applying thumb walking technique. When starting work on a foot, you are testing to see what level of pressure is appropriate, in general, for the individual's foot. Start lightly and adjust pressure according to the response you get. Some feet will respond only to light pressure throughout the session.

Light pressure in itself can be utilized purely as a relaxation technique. Light pressure application can also provide a quick evaluation of the foot to generally gauge touch stress cues in an area, region, or the whole foot.

Medium pressure

Medium pressure describes a moderate level of challenge used with a foot that shows signs of the adaptation stage. A lack of visual stress cues, a general consistent thickness throughout the foot, and/or moderate sensitivity to technique application call for a level of technique application that challenges the foot moderately. It is a level of pressure that you will find works effectively with almost anyone, and it is the level of pressure you will be working with most of the time. "It hurts good" is a comment frequently heard in reference to this level of pressure.

Heavy pressure

Heavy pressure describes an upper range of challenge utilized for the highly adapted foot. Callousing or thick, heavy feet with no sensitivity or feet that have been conditioned by the application of moderate pressure over time call for technique application of a sufficient magnitude to cause a response. Heavy pressure may be appropriate when medium pressure does not seem to bring a response.

Heavy pressure is not a beginning level pressure. It is not appropriate for all individuals. However, some individuals prefer a more vigorous workout and they may request more pressure. For these individuals, a heavy level of pressure "hurts good."

Take care not to overstress your own thumb. The leverage of the working hand is particularly important in applying this level of pressure. Also, be aware of the effect your technique application has on the individual. Sensitivity levels will change during the course of a session. You may find a sudden breakthrough where a previously insensitive area is suddenly sensitive.

Frequency of Passes

The frequency of passes of pressure techniques over a particular area is gauged by the amount of pressure you are using. The lighter the pressure, the more frequent the passes needed to achieve a conditioning effect.

Five to ten passes of thumb walking technique are sufficient to assess an area for stress cues or to apply medium or heavy pressure.

5 to 10 Passes

By applying ten to fifteen passes you are conditioning the foot with light to medium pressure.

10 to 15 Passes

Fifteen or more passes show special attention to a stressed area that calls for light pressure. If you are applying 15 to 20 passes of medium to heavy pressure, consider other technique strategies.

15 to 20 Passes

Where to Apply Technique

Noting where to apply technique is a part of the reflexologist's strategy. For the most part you will apply technique, however, in some instances avoiding an area or working around it or working from several directions is the best strategy.

Approach is an initial and gradual introduction of pressure to the foot. You are gauging the individual's likes, dislikes and any extreme sensitivity. When the individual comments "That feels good," note the technique you are using and/or the part of the foot being worked. The area can be used as the individual's relaxation area, somewhat akin to the solar plexus area – as an overall area of relaxation. It may just feel good to the individual or it may be an indicator of a key area or technique likely to cause a change in a stress pattern and/or mechanism.

Strategy one: Approach

Avoidance is a technique procedure for noting the technique or parts of the foot to which the individual responds negatively. Most frequently this will be a response of extreme sensitivity. The individual reports that "It hurts bad" or "I don't like that."

Strategy two: Avoidance

Working the surrounding area is a technique strategy utilized to work with stress cues such as extreme sensitivity, sensitivity that increases rather than decreases with work, corns, and sensitive callousing. To apply the technique procedure, apply technique to the area adjacent to the area of sensitivity, gradually working closer and closer to the area of interest. Thus, you work within the individual's comfort zone and indirectly work the area.

Strategy three: Working the surrounding area

115

Working the surrounding area is also utilized rather than repeatedly applying thumb walking technique to a stressed area and possibly overworking it. It provides a break in technique application to an area of interest and allows time for the foot to adapt and create a change in the stress pattern.

**Strategy four:
Working from
several directions**

The goal of this technique procedure is to gather more information and to provide variety to the stressed area. Once a part of the foot has drawn your attention through observation of a stress cue, approach the area of interest from several viewpoints. Thumb walking technique applied from several different directions provides a depth to your assessment and technique application. The stress cue may be apparent from one directional approach but not another. Sensitivity may be elicited from working one direction and not another. The individual may even report that one particular directional approach feels "good" and thus better than other approaches.

**Strategy five:
Note any change**

Noting any change allows you to focus on the effects of your technique application. Is there any change in the size, shape or dimensions of the stress cue in response to your work? Consider the area under your thumb after a few passes. Consider a region of the foot after some work. Finally, consider the whole foot after technique application. **Remember the Basic Rule of Change within the Stress Pattern. The more quickly change occurs in response to pressure, the less the impact of the stress, the shorter the duration of time it has been there, and the less time required to condition the foot**.

**Strategy six:
Encourage self-help**

Self-help techniques are applied by the client between sessions. At time, your work is not enough to break up the pattern of stress sufficiently. The value of self-help is twofold: It encourages individuals to get involved in their own health, and it speeds up results. Your client may or may not be interested in learning everything about reflexology or the techniques, but he or she may be interested in an appropriate self-help technique or two. Choose your objectives. Target only a limited number of areas for your client to work on, because self-help homework can be confusing and unusable if not clearly and simply defined. For further information, see Kunz and Kunz, *Reflexology, Health at your fingertips*, Dorling Kindersly, 2003 or Kunz and Kunz, *Hand And Foot Reflexology, A Self-Help Guide*, New York, Simon and Schuster, 1984.

Number of Sessions

How many sessions will be required to cause a change sufficient to meet the individual's goal(s)? The stimulus of pressure interrupts stress and evokes a response of relaxation within a single session. The actual number of

Foot Relaxation Scale

The amount and type of work necessary to condition a foot stress cue is shown on the Foot Relaxation Scale. The left-hand column lists technique strategy, the work necessary to create change in the stress level. The next three columns list various levels of stress adaptation. Consider the technique strategy listed as appropriate for each level of stress adaptation. Try the various technique strategies to note the change that takes place in stress patterns. The goal of technique strategy is to create predictable change.

Technique Strategy	Alarm	Adaptation	Exhaustion
	Puffiness; sensitivity; some white speckling; foot feature	Thickness; white speckling; prominent foot feature; sharp/deep sensitivity; streaks of red/white; white bumps	Callousing; extreme puffiness, foot feature, or sensitivity; hard tonus; sheets of red/white; raised white bumps
Amount of Pressure			
Light	infant's foot	to test stress cues	older foot
Medium	after conditioning has taken place	√ (moderately adapted)	after education has taken place
Heavy		√ (highly adapted)	callousing
Number of passes			
5 to 10	assess an area	assess an area	assess an area
10 to 15	conditioning with light pressure	conditioning with medium pressure	conditioning with light pressure
15 to 20	special attention with light pressure	conditioning with medium pressure	special attention with light pressure
Number of sessions			
Interrupting stress	any one session	any one session	any one session
Conditioning stress	two to four sessions	four to eight sessions with maintenance	eight or more sessions with maintenance
Educating stress	four to eight sessions with maintenance	eight or more sessions with maintenance	

sessions necessary to achieve a goal varies from individual to individual. What is predictable is that change will take place. What is unpredictable is whether or not it will be enough to meet the individual's goals.

Interrupting stress response

The goal of interrupting stress takes place during any one session. Most individuals experience a feeling of relaxation all over the body. The individual who does not experience a relaxation effect immediately will require three to five sessions to break the established pattern of stress. Many individuals report a change in their perception of their feet. They will often state that they didn't realize their feet could feel so relaxed, that their feet feel lighter, or that they feel their feet are in better contact with the ground.

Conditioning stress response

Technique application over several sessions conditions the foot and creates a change in overall stress pattern. A conditioning effect should take place with sessions once or twice a week over a two to four week period. The individual who initially experienced adaptive stress cues should report that an alleviation of stress-related symptoms has taken place and spans a progressively longer time period, for example, for two days following the session to four days to a week. Once the improvement in symptoms spans from session to session, some ongoing technique application will be needed to maintain and up-keep the conditioning effect. A session every two weeks or once a month with some self-help should maintain the level of conditioning.

Educating stress response

Ongoing work educates the foot to respond to stress in the best possible manner. With four to eight weeks of technique application, the individual who initially experienced deeply ingrained stress cues should report a more lasting effect. Education has taken place when little or no sensitivity is reported and many of the adapted stress cues show change. On-going technique application every two weeks or once a month with self-help will maintain and up-keep the conditioning effect.

Variables

A very ill person may respond immediately to technique application. Any lessening of the individual's stressed and exhausted state can create dramatic contrast. Ironically, less technique application may be required to create a change with the very sick or chronically ill individual.

Consider it a "stubborn" stress response when the individual reports little change from session to session. This individual may have a hard time relaxing and may be conditioned to an overall high tension level. More technique application is needed over a longer period of time to condition and create a change. Make a goal of reducing the overall stress level. Consider a session with multiple desserts and light pressure applied to the solar plexus reflex area and the individual's key stress cues.

Interviewing the Client

Your verbal interaction with the client is an important part of any session. In talking to the owner of the foot before, during, and after your session, you are gathering more information, giving an assessment, and, overall, demonstrating your professional competence. The interview is a focused, systematic effort to communicate your findings and to elicit the individual's feelings.

Some individuals will immediately tell you what you need to know about their stress level. This individual will comment on his or her stress history, goals for your work with him or her, and his or her perception of your work as it progresses. Other individuals will need prompting to describe their feelings. Either way, you will want a consistent, systematic method to interview the individual. The interview during the session tells you what stress factors and relaxation goals are present. This information combined with your findings will determine how much conditioning and what type will be required to relax the individual's stress pattern.

The interview includes listening, asking questions, and being observant of verbal cues. You want to get the person talking. Asking questions focuses the individual on his or her stress pattern and goals. In addition, a casual yet systematic interview focuses your work on developing a session custom tailored for that individual.

Stress History

The individual's feet in front of you are a history of who the individual is, what he or she has been doing, and how long he or she has been doing it. To respond with a session that is just right, the reflexologist considers the individual's preset level of tension. The starting point for your work is, in essence, the individual's overall level of background tension. The preset tension level includes the exposure of the individual's foot and body to use, overuse, illness, and/or injury.

Time is a factor that indicates how long a particular stress has affected the individual. How old is the individual? How much time has he or she spent or is spending at a standing, sitting, stressful, or physical occupation? Does the individual play sports or engage in a hobby activity that places stresses on his or her body or results in frequent injury. How many injuries, car accidents, major illnesses, and so forth has the individual experienced and at what age? How long has it been since an injury or stressful event

Age Comparison

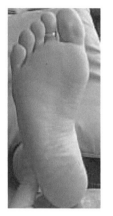

Daughter: 17

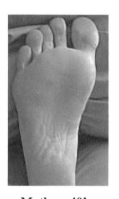

Mother: 40's

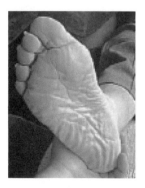

Grandmother: 70's

occurred? This information is important to the reflexologist in planning his or her session. Remember, the longer something has been adapted to, the greater the possibility that it has become established as a stress pattern. It follows that the more serious the stress event and/or the more stress events or injuries at a younger age, the more complex the stress pattern.

The stress history portion of the interview allows you to note the impact of past and current stress by gathering information about age, heredity, occupation, and stress events. **The Basic Rule of a Stress History is (1) The older the individual, (2) the longer the time since the stress event, (3) the greater the impact of the stress or stress event, (4) the more time spent in a sitting or standing or walking occupation or physical occupation, (5) the more time wearing impractical shoes, the greater the chance for ingrained wear-and-tear patterns and injury and the more technique application will be required to interrupt, condition, or educate the stress mechanism.**

Age

Selye considered the stages of adaptation to be analogous with the stages of life. Childhood compared to the alarm stage because of the learning aspects of both; adult ages paralleled the adaptation stage; older ages compared to the exhaustion phase of adaptation.

Children and young adults are still growing. Because children's bodies have yet to fully establish a response to stress, patterns of stress are not deeply ingrained. Thus, you can expect to observe lesser stress cues, perhaps sharp areas that respond quickly to technique application, and, in general, quicker changes than are observable in an adult.

The older the person, obviously, the greater the potential for deeply ingrained stress patterns, as there is a greater potential for past stress events such as injury. In general, it may be more difficult to interrupt stress and to maintain the interruption. In turn, the more stress cues you observe and the older the individual, the less aggressive the approach you should take. Applying challenging techniques to an exhausted foot may elicit more exhaustion.

Stress and Stress Coping Mechanisms

To get an idea about the individual's perception of his or her health and stress level, ask a neutral question such as, "Are you in pretty good health?"

Such a question will usually elicit a response that indicates whether the person perceives his or her body to be under stress and in what manner.

Asking a question such as, "Do you take pretty good care of yourself?" tells you how the person copes with stress. Such a question will typically elicit information about activities such as seeking medical help regularly, visiting the health spa frequently, taking vitamins, paying attention to diet and health habits, working out at home, or visiting a massage therapist, acupuncturist, or other therapist.

Heredity

Hereditary factors are important because they contribute to your future expectations and the client's. It is not only the stress of a lifetime that is reflected in the feet before you but also reflected are hereditary factors of general health, foot structure and stress coping mechanisms. Hereditary factors may not be easy to ascertain in a stress history. Listen for clues as to family health patterns.

Occupation

Work, especially standing, walking, and physically active occupations (e.g., waitress, salesclerk, factory worker) creates particular stresses for the foot and body. Signs of foot overuse and adaptation are common in standing occupations. The longer the workday and the more years on the feet, the greater the potential for fatigue throughout the foot. Additional stresses can be created by standing in a fixed position and/or the wearing of high heels.

Sitting occupations create a unique range of stresses. The more hours a day that one is seated and the more stationary the position, the greater the potential for general body fatigue. The feet may tend to show fewer signs of adaptation than standing feet; however, they tend to reflect a lack of muscle tone.

Physical occupations such as construction and assembly work offer the potential for injury and overuse in addition to the stress of standing and walking. The foot shows signs of adaptation and fatigue.

Stress Event

In response to a stress cue of note, a question such as, "Have you ever injured yourself?" will tell you how much stress the individual faces due to

Standing Occupation

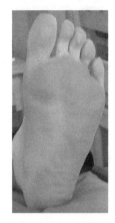

• **Stress cues: flat foot, extreme red coloring along the pattern of pressure sensors typical to a foot during standing.**
• **Occupation: Medical doctor**

Stress Event

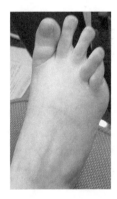

• **Stress cue: extreme position of toes**
• **Question: "Have you ever injured yourself?"**
• **Answer: "Yes, a serious car accident resulting in whiplash."**

121

Hobby

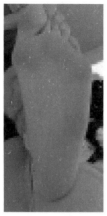

- **Stress cue: extreme callousing, toe positions**
- **Hobby: triathlete**

past stress events. Trauma to the body is reflected as a stress experience observable on the foot. Take note of the report of any stress events such as a car accident, an operation, a high school sports-related injury, a major illness, or an on-the-job injury. How serious was the event and how long ago did it happen? These two questions provide a picture of how ingrained the stress adaptation has become.

In response to a stress cue of note, especially in the solar plexus reflex area, you might also ask, "Do you feel as if you are under stress?" Frequently the individual will respond with a report about stress at home or at the workplace.

Ultimately, the reflexologist targets the root cause of the health concern. For some, it's a hereditary pattern, for others it's occupational stress, for still others it's an accident or illness, that, added to a level of on-going stress, creates a pattern.

Sports and Hobby Activities

Leisure time activities can produce stress for the body. Tennis, for example, creates over-work for the ball of the feet. It is not unusual for marathon runners to report foot pain.

Stress History and the Reflex Relaxation Scale

The existing stress patterns do have an impact on how long it will take to create change. Age tells you how long the individual has accumulated the stress patterns. Stress events tell you what reflex patterns have been set up in response to accidents, injuries, and emotional distress.

In asking the question, How long will it take to create change? the learning curve in regard to conditioning reflexes is considered. Each stage of adaptation is evaluated in light of the stress history of the individual. When observing, for example, the feet of a young adult which show signs of exhaustion, consider the possibility that this person may have experienced a major stress event in his or her life. Thus, the amount of technique application to create change will be greater than that required for a young adult without the major stress event. The individual's stress history has a direct impact on their stage of adaptation. Stress history provides predictable elements that allow you to estimate the amount of technique application necessary to create a change in the reflex stress pattern.

Alarm: An alarm reflex pattern is not yet etched into the body's reflexive patterns. Children and individuals of any age with a recent injury, a recent stress, or a recent standing occupation may be in this category.

Adaptation: Adult, or an individual of any age with a one to five year time period since injury, major stress, or in a standing occupation.

Exhaustion: Older adult OR an individual of any age with a recent major injury, illness, operation, or stress, OR an individual with an injury or a stress that occurred five or more years ago, OR an individual in a standing occupation for five or more years.

Reflex Relaxation Scale

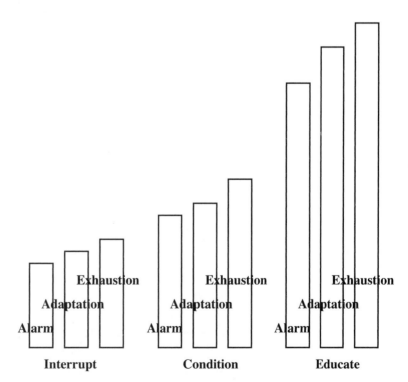

Stress History
Older adult or individual: • with a recent major illness or injury,   • in a standing occupation for five or more years, or   • who experienced the injury or major stress five or more years ago.
Any individual: • with a recent major illness, injury, or stress,   • in a standing occupation for one to five years, or   • who experienced the injury or major stress one to five years ago.
Child or any individual: • with a current or recent stress   • injury or   • with a recent standing occupation

Interrupt   Condition   Educate

Alarm   Adaptation   Exhaustion (×3)

**Amount of work (Technique application)
Necessary to create change (Relaxation)**

Eliciting Relaxation Goals and the Body Relaxation Scale

Most individuals have some sort of goal in mind when visiting a reflexologist. It is a part of the reflexologist's role to elicit and recognize goal statements from the individual. It is also a part of the reflexologist's role to consider whether or not the individual's expectations are realistic. These are skills developed by focusing on communication with the individual: listening, asking questions, and being observant in general to verbal cues. Such information helps you decide on which stress cues to focus.

At the start of a session, asking a question will give you a general idea of what the individual is seeking to accomplish through the use of reflexology. "What exactly are you looking for in reflexology?" or "Have you had your feet worked on before?" are questions that help create a focus for your session.

Consider the individual's response or general comment about goals. What, in general, is the individual signaling as a stress reduction goal? Is it a foot stress goal? Or is it a reflex stress goal? Is it a body goal or a combination of goals? Once the individual has indicated what part of the stress pattern he or she is interested in relaxing, consider the end result the person would like to see.

Typical comments or responses about stress patterns include:

Foot stress goals (tired feet): "Ever since I got this new pair of shoes, my feet have been killing me." "My feet hurt." "I work on my feet all day." "I'm aware of the tension in my feet all the time."

Foot stress goals (foot problem, operation, injury): "I've had a foot operation, injury, and/or foot problem and I want to take better care of my feet." (*Note*: The reflexologist does not work with any foot problem that is undiagnosed.)

Reflex stress goal (stress-related condition, operation, injury): "My shoulder bothers me." "My digestion bothers me." "I've heard reflexology could help with back problems." "My back bothers me all the time." "I've had surgery on my eyes." "I had a car accident six months ago." (*Note:* The reflexologist does not work with any undiagnosed or specific problem.)

Body stress goal (relaxation, stress reduction): "I've been stressed at home/work. I'm looking for anything to reduce my stress level."

Typical comments or responses about desired results include:

Prevention: "I'm interested in taking care of myself. I'd rather spend the money now to relax tension than later to pay medical bills."

Maintenance: "I like to do good things for my health."

Touch: "I'm single and I treat myself to these little luxuries."

Awareness: "I like having my feet worked on."

Performance: "I just don't feel that good any more." "I know I'm pushing my body, but I have deadlines to meet."

Body Relaxation Scale

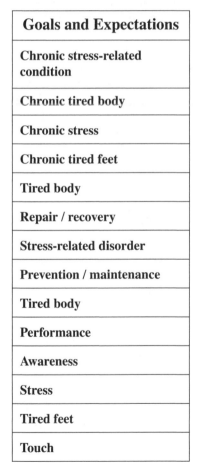

Goals and Expectations
Chronic stress-related condition
Chronic tired body
Chronic stress
Chronic tired feet
Tired body
Repair / recovery
Stress-related disorder
Prevention / maintenance
Tired body
Performance
Awareness
Stress
Tired feet
Touch

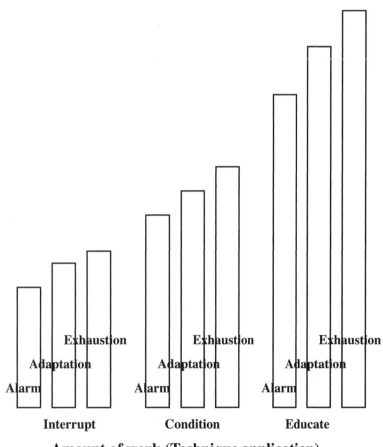

Interrupt   Condition   Educate

(Exhaustion / Adaptation / Alarm)

Amount of work (Technique application)
Necessary to create change (Relaxation)

Matching Expectations

Now that the individual has told you his or her feelings and goals, consider your findings. A goal of relaxing tired feet, for example, is considered in relationship to the foot you are observing. How much stress is present in the foot and how much of a conditioning effect does the individual want to achieve? This will dictate the amount of technique application that will be required to reach the goal.

It is important to remember: (1) Some goals require more work than others, (2) Some goals are more ambitious than others, (3) Some goals require a shift in response to stress by the individual. What is realistically possible for the individual?

Any goal statement is a request for interruption of stress. Once you have applied technique and interrupted stress during a session, you would expect the individual to feel some relaxation of the stress. The individual, however, may also be seeking a longer lasting effect. Does the individual want his or her tired feet to feel better when walking out of your office after one session? Does the individual want his or her tired feet to feel better between sessions, for a week at a time? Or is the individual looking for a long-range solution to tired feet?

The skill comes from listening and considering what is possible for this individual with your session. It may not be easy to interrupt the stress pattern of, for example, a foot that is in the exhaustion stage of adaptation. It is important to match the individual's stage of adaptation with what can realistically be expected from the session. To match the individual's expectations with your findings, ask yourself, What is the likely response to the application of technique?

Interrupting stress: Is your expectation of the results of technique application that the individual will feel lessened stress after one session and that perhaps the feeling will last a few days?

Conditioning stress: Is your expectation of the results of technique application that the individual will feel lessened stress that will last between sessions, say a week or longer?

Educating stress: Is your expectation that the feeling of lessened stress will be continuous with some maintenance and that the individual may move on to some new goals?

Observing and Noting Changes in Stress Response

How do you know if you have reached your goal of creating a change in the individual's stress mechanism? Also, how does the client know that he or she has received something of value through the application of reflexology technique? Changes in tension level are observable. By observing and noting changes, the reflexologist provides himself or herself as well as the client with an opportunity to make an ongoing stress history to gauge response to technique application. Over the long term, progress toward the individual's goals can be measured. During the course of a session, you will observe and note changes in response to technique application, changes in the appearance of stress cues, in sensitivity, and in comments from the client.

Change in the foot stress mechanism is gauged by asking questions during the session. The answers will tell you how quickly and how much change took place in response to technique application. During the session, point out changes in the stress cues. For example, note, "This area is less puffy than it was." Or ask, "Is that area (a previously sensitive area, for example) as sensitive as it was?" "How does your foot feel?" "This area feels less pronounced to me. How does it feel to you?"

Note the individual's comments during the session. "My headache feels better." "I can't feel the tension between my shoulder blades any more." "I'm so relaxed I could fall asleep."

After work on one foot, ask the individual, "Would you mind getting up and taking a few steps? Now, do you feel a difference between the two feet?" The individual's response gives you feedback about how quickly he or she is responding (or is not responding) to your work. Answers range from "It feels like a new foot" to "It feels like a pillow" to "It's okay" to "It feels better than it did" to "It feels about the same."

At the finish of your work, ask, "How does that feel?" prompts the individual to note the effects of your work. Typical comments that gauge the response to the session include: "That feels better." (Indication that some interruption of stress has taken place.) "That feels great" or "That feels like a whole new foot." (Indication that interruption of stress has taken place.)

At the start of the next session ask, "How do you feel?" The individual will probably make a general response such as, "I feel pretty good" or "I feel about the same." A follow-up question to elicit more information is a statement and question such as "You felt pretty good at the end of the previous session. How long did that feeling last?" The individual's responses allow you to note any change in the overall stress mechanism. The individual who reports, "I felt good a few days after the last session" is signaling that, although stress was interrupted, the foot is not yet conditioned to a lesser stage of stress adaptation. The individual who reports, "I felt good the entire time between sessions" is signaling that conditioning has taken place. The individual who says, "I didn't even notice the stress condition this week" has reached an educated stage of adaptation. The level of response is a reflection of change in stress pattern following technique application.

With each session during the series, consider the ongoing progress of the stress pattern. Signs of a lasting improvement include, "I can stand all day and my feet don't bother me any more" or "My feet feel like a million dollars" or "I suddenly realized I could turn my head in traffic without turning my whole body – my neck is doing so much better" or "I just plain feel better" or "I was under a lot of stress last week with work and I could handle it."

The Session Plan

Planning

Work with the client to create a plan of action to reduce his or her stress. A certain amount of technique application will be required to create the change he or she is seeking. To clarify the commitment necessary to achieve goals, discuss the amount of adaptation present and the amount of technique application required under the circumstances.

To match the individual's expectations with what you have observed on the feet, consider that the goal of reflexology is to provide relaxation and, over time, a conditioning effect. It is a basic tenet of reflexology that an adequate supply of technique application will cause a change in the stress mechanism. The more the adaptation to stress, the more the alteration of brain-organ dynamics and the more the application of technique required to create change.

The goal of the individual should be to apply pressure technique sufficient to teach the body a better adaptation to stress. The individual utilizes the services of the reflexologist and self-help as a tool to meet goals. Ask yourself if the individual has set realistic goals. For example, does the individual expect to reverse a lifetime of stress adaptations in one session? The reflexologist works to create a realistic goal by clarifying the amount of effort necessary to achieve the potential goal.

Give the individual a general evaluation of the stress and stress level you have observed in his or her feet. Include a general idea of your perspective of how much reflexology work would be appropriate and needed for his or her stress pattern. Your comments are framed in reference to the stage of adaptation and the wear-and-tear pattern you have observed. You give the individual an indication of his or her starting point stage of adaptation to suggest the extent of the technique application that will be required to cause a change. You want to apprise the individual about how much commitment will be needed on his or her part to reach the relaxation goal.

An example of such as approach is, "I see quite a few signs of adaptation (stress cues) that have been here for a while. The pattern of stress cues and your answers to questions seem to indicate that the pattern of stress has become a recurring problem to you. While you have experienced a few major stress events in the recent past, you have indicated that you have made an effort to take care of yourself. It will require regular technique application to achieve the goal of maintenance that you have indicated. I can do part of that and you can do part of that through self-help techniques."

Possible comments that can be used to signal your appraisal include:
• **Occasional stress** "I see a few signs of stress. Your feet seem to be in pretty good overall shape. It shouldn't take a long time to condition these feet."
•**Recurring, moderate stress** "I see a fair amount of stress cues but, overall, the foot seems to be in good shape. It will take a moderate amount of technique application to destress these feet. You can speed up the process and keep up with the stress level through self-help.
• **Chronic stress** "I see quite a few stress cues that have been here for quite a while. It will take a while to condition these feet, but you can help speed the process with self–help."

The S. O. A. P. P. Formula

You've observed the foot, assessed the foot, and had discussions with your client. What you've been doing is gathering information appropriate to a reflexological appraisal of the foot. It's also information suitable for an assessment format standard to the medical profession. Whether or not you work with medical personnel, the S. O. A. P. P. Formula will help you organize your work.

The S. O. A. P. P. Formula is a standard format for evaluating and communicating information between medical personnel. S. O. A. P. P. is an abbreviation for:
• **Subjective** information, the client's viewpoint
• **Objective** information, what the reflexologist observes and feels with his or her hands
• **Assessment,** the reflexologist's evaluation of the situation in terms of his or her profession, the why's and how's of what has been observed
• **Plan,** the reflexologist's estimation of a future program of action for the client: improvement possibilities, specific identified techniques, and number of sessions over a period of time
• **Preventive**, the reflexologist's suggestions for preventing future occurrences.

The S. O. A. P. P. Formula is both a comprehensive assessment procedure and a completed document form. It forms the basis for an effective series of sessions for the client. The S. O. A. P. P. Formula conveys information from a specialist about information gathered from the client as well as the practitioner's observations of assessment and plan of action for a client in the terms of the specialty field. See p. 229 for an example.

Subjective Information

Subjective information is gathered from what the client feels, desires, and requires. It consists of client comments about his or her feelings and perceptions about general and specific existing health states. As noted in the section "Interviewing the Client," the reflexologist notes, listens and elicits comments about the client's stress history including: general well-being, client's evaluation of general health, client's attempts to work towards health betterment, client's feelings about state of health, and causative factors that resulted in state of health.

Other relevant factors of stress history are considered as well: age (general), occupation / approximate number of years, hobbies / sports participation / approximate number of years, stress / stress event (past and current), foot injury (when), injury or accident (when), major illness (when).

Objective Information

The reflexologist gathers information about what he or she observes when assessing the feet. As noted in "Assessing the Foot," this is accomplished during hands-on work: with: stress cue observations (visual, touch, press and assess, sensitivity); client comments about technique application; client answers to relevant questions are noted: "Does your, e. g. neck, bother you?"

Assessment

Observations are evaluated to analyze the how's and why's of the client's stress pattern in reflexological terms. Inferences are drawn from stress cue observations. Such inferences are noted in "Assessing the Foot" and include:

Foot stress inferences: Considering the stress cues and stages of adaptation (alarm, adaptation or exhaustion) and making a qualitative assessment of observed stress cues, i. e. compared to other feet, is this the hardest tonus I have observed?

Reflex stress inferences: Considering the location, type (alarm, adapted and exhausted), and number of stress cues; consider the appropriateness of the stress cues in light of the individual's stress history and age.

Body stress inferences: Evaluating body stress cues and the reflections on the body as well as client response to questions.

Plan

The reflexologist's plan apprises the client and/or medical personnel about the proposed reflexology plan of action needed to reach the client's goals. Client comments about goals are included. In reference to foot reflexology work, common goals are to work with: Health problem or injury, health maintenance / prevention goal, relaxation of over-used or tired feet, foot injury, body awareness, physical touch, stress reduction, pain reduction

Compare the individual's goals to the stress cue observations and inferences. Consider the improvement possibilities. Then, the reflexologist determines a strategy consisting of: Types of technique application and targeted reflex areas (foot relaxation); Number of sessions / targeted reflex areas (reflex relaxation); Goal of technique application (body relaxation).

Prevention

The reflexologist considers preventive measures such as shoe wear, surface commonly underfoot, and self-help technique suggestions.

The Session Procedure

The following is a step-by-step description of proceeding through a session. A systematic procedure allows you to concentrate your efforts on the individual because it frees you to emphasize technique application appropriate to that individual. Finally, an organized, consistent approach adds to your professional image.

1 Prepare your workplace.

Wash your hands. Check your fingernail length. Check your workplace for cleanliness and neatness.

2 Begin your session.

Your session begins when the client enters the room. Observe walking, body position and shoes. Invite the individual to sit and remove his or her shoes and socks.

3 Look over the entire foot.

Ask the individual if there is any part of the foot that should be avoided, such as injured areas, cuts, bruises, rashes, infections, ingrown nails. Make sure any wound or break in the skin is covered. Look for the extreme stress cue that may indicate a part of the foot that should be approached carefully or avoided altogether. A red, angry bunion; a corn; a plantar wart; split skin between toes; cracked callousing; athlete's foot; and foot problems that need the attention of a podiatrist all fall in this category.

4 Begin work with a series of desserts.

You, thus, warm up the foot and prepare it for technique application. A cold foot or a foot lacking in circulation may respond with more sensitivity. Make a preliminary assessment of visual stress cues. Consider your general impression of the foot, the most outstanding visual stress cues, and their locations.

5 Ask a general question about goals.

Ask a question, such as, "Have you ever had your feet done before?" or "Are you familiar with reflexology?" or "Why did you decide to try reflexology?" At this point it may be necessary to clarify the nature of your service. If the individual is seeking medical services, note that you cannot treat for a specific illness. If the individual is experiencing an acute or undiagnosed problem, refer him or her to the appropriate medical services.

6 Consider appropriate level of pressure.

Begin your work with a level of pressure appropriate to the individual. A thin adult foot, an older foot, a younger foot, or a foot very sensitive to initial contact call for a light touch. A heavy foot may require a heavy pressure to register a sensation.

7 Apply technique.

As you work through the feet, adjust your pressure level by watching the individual's facial response to your work. To stay within the individual's comfort zone, ask the individual to tell you when the pressure of technique application is too much.

In most cases this will be the holding hand because you will constantly be repositioning the working hand to work other areas. Your thumb or fingers may get tired. Learn how to vary your techniques to avoid fatigue. For example, when the walking thumb begins to tire, change to a dessert, or switch hands and walk with the other thumb from the opposite direction. As you build your hand strength over a period of time, this will be less of a concern.

8 Keep at least one hand on the foot.

Follow a systematic, repeatable pattern to work through the foot. (See Suggested Session Pattern, pp. 64-65.) Make an assessment of the touch stress cues as you work. Consider the characteristics and location of the stress cues. Make a press and assess evaluation of any part of the foot that draws your interest. Compare the stress cues in the toes to those in the ball of the foot and other parts of the foot. Note sensitivity reported by the individual. Compare the touch cues to the visual cues. Gather information about the individual's perception of his or her stress.

9 Follow systematic pattern of technique application and assessment.

After you work through the foot for the first time, select areas of emphasis for technique application during the second time through the foot. Consider the pattern of technique application that would be most appropriate to relax the observed stress cues.

10 Consider your evaluation of the foot.

Work through the foot a second time, making a more detailed assessment of the areas of interest and the general pattern of stress. Note any change in the stress cue as technique is applied and after technique is applied. Consider whether any of the selected areas is more relaxed (i.e., a puffy area is less puffy, a thickened area is less thick). Apply a series of desserts to finish your work on the foot. Consider whether or not the foot feels more relaxed than it did during the initial series of desserts.

11 Work through the foot a second time targeting selected areas of emphasis.

Ask the individual to get up and take a few steps to compare and contrast one foot with the other. Note the response to your work on the one foot.

12 Ask individual to take a few steps.

Repeat the above procedures, working with the other foot. Compare this foot to the first foot. Did you find similar stress cues? A similar overall feel to the foot? Widely different stress cues? More sensitivity?

13 Work through the other foot.

At the end of the session, ask the individual to participate with you in a breathing exercise. The breathing exercise is used to finish a session and to focus attention on his or her overall relaxation level. To practice the breathing exercise, place the flats of the thumbs on the bottoms of the feet in the solar plexus area. Ask the individual to take four deep breaths along with you

14 Ask individual to participate in breathing exercise.

as you exert a constant steady pressure with both thumbs. On the last exhalation of breath, gradually remove the thumbs from the surfaces of the feet.

15 Ask a general question.

Ask a general question such as, "What do you think?" or "How do you feel?" to gauge the individual's response to technique application.

16 Consider results of your work.

Consider how much change took place and how quickly in response to your work. Consider the overall stress level of the feet and the stress history of the individual. Compare the individual's rate of response to your expectations for similar patterns of stress such as age or stage of adaptation. Note whether or not change took place at the rate you expected.

17 Create a session plan for the individual.

Outline the responses you observed and an assessment of the overall stress pattern. Give the individual an estimation of how much reflexology work will be required to achieve the goal that he or she has indicated.

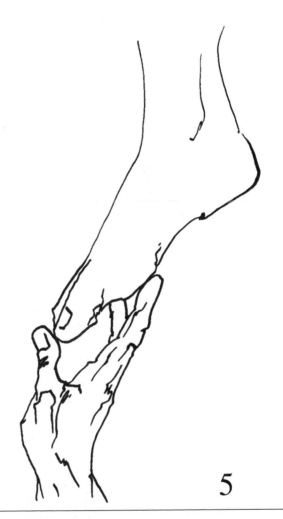

You the Reflexologist

You, the Reflexologist

The reflexologist is a professional and a business person. Success in both areas calls for particular skills. A successful professional is not merely skillful. The practice of professional reflexology requires a systematic approach and the self-discipline to act within the standards of a professional field. A reflexologist acts within the defined boundaries in order to receive increased respect and remuneration. Among skills for success in business are an understanding of how to organize and run a service provider business.

Reflexology Professionalism

Any professional plays a particular role in society. The professional model defines that role. A professional has received training in and has achieved a mastery over a particular body of knowledge. The community sanctions the practice of the specialist because of this refined knowledge. In addition, the professional signals concern for public safety issues involving the practice by following standards and practices appropriate to the specialty.

As a reflexologist, you signal your professionalism through what you say, do, and display in the workplace. What you say and do demonstrates you mastery of professional skills. You want the individual to feel safe in your hands, that you are well qualified, and that this is a service he or she values. Preparation is required to reflect a credible professional image. In reflexology this includes the consideration of basic professional issues.

Reflexologist Defined

A reflexologist applies pressure techniques to the feet or hands with the goal of exercising pressure sensors. The reflexologist has the ability to select the appropriate technique for the area of the foot or hand and to apply the technique with maximum efficiency and effect. He or she has the ability to assess the foot or hand in terms of zones and reflex areas. He or she has the ability to select stressed areas on the foot (or hand) that require technique application. The reflexologist has the ability to describe the workings of reflexology within the nervous system. The reflexologist knows about and provides services within the professional standards and practices of the field.

The reflexologist makes an assessment in the terms of the belief system, reflexology. The purpose of the reflexologist in his or her conversation with the individual is to make an assessment of the foot and its stress cues.

The reflexologist asks questions to determine whether his or her measurement of stress matches that of the individual. It is not the goal of the reflexologist to tell the individual what is wrong with him or her. The reflexologist acts to relax the foot and body by application of pressure techniques determined by an evaluation of the stress cues.

Standards and Practices

The reflexologist provides specialized services within ethical boundaries. These boundaries are the rules and guidelines that define the standards and practices of the field. The standards and practices of reflexology have evolved in response to professional concerns and community requests to define the specialized service. Questions about consumer safety, professional safeguards, the uniqueness of services, and ethical-legal standards are areas of concern to governmental bodies seeking to protect the public. Ultimately the parameters of the profession are balanced with the needs of the community to create a professional service. What follows is a discussion of the standards and practices of the field of reflexology.

Professional Boundaries

Business licensing is required of businesses in most cities. The general issue is one of taxation and zoning. Not all businesses are allowed to operate in any zoned area. To ascertain business licensing and zoning requirements, contact the appropriate department of the city government, usually the taxation and revenue department.

Business licensing

In some cities and states of the United States, the provider of reflexology services is required to obtain reflexology or massage therapy licensing. To ascertain licensing requirements, contact the appropriate department of the city government, usually the taxation and revenue department, or the state professional regulation and licensing department.

Professional licensing

Professions are licensed for many reasons among them to protect the public from untrained individuals. Using the vocabulary of another profession or providing services licensed to another profession are issues of concern. Concerns include work applied by the reflexologist that could be construed as infringing on the licensed professions of:

Infringing on other licensed professions

Medicine: diagnosis, prescription or treating for a specific illness
Massage: work applied to any part of the body other than the hands and feet
Chiropractics: "adjustment" of the feet or hands
Podiatry: treating diseases of the feet.

HIPAA   Under certain circumstances, the reflexologist is subject to The Health Insurance Portability and Accountability Act (HIPAA). HIPAA was enacted by Congress in 1996. In addition to other provisions, HIPAA security and privacy standards assure consumers that their personal health information will be protected from inappropriate uses and disclosures.

Contra-indications to reflexology work   Do not apply reflexology work to (1) any part of the foot that shows observable trauma or possibility of pain, (2) an injured area, (3) an ingrown nail, (4) a cut, (5) a red, angry bunion, (6) a bruise, (7) a corn, (8) a rash, (9) a plantar wart, (10) infection, (11) a split skin between toes, (12) athlete's foot, (13) callousing that is cracked, (14) any foot problem that requires the attention of a podiatrist.

Further contra indications include: (1) any undiagnosed health problem, (2) any problem that needs medical attention – persistent pain or a chronic medical problem that gets worse, (3) any problem about which the individual reports urgent concern.

Reflexology is a safe practice if used properly. The reflexologist should always be aware of pacing his or her work according to the individual. Working with an individual who reports diabetes, hypoglycemia, unstable pregnancy, extreme age, or extreme illness requires an awareness that you are applying technique to an individual with special needs. If in doubt, request a medical opinion before proceeding with your work.

When to make a medical referral   Never hesitate to make a medical referral and/or ask a physician's permission before proceeding with your reflexology services. Any individual who indicates that he or she is seeking your services in lieu of medical services should be referred to a physician immediately. In addition, do not work with an individual who reports an undiagnosed physical problem. Working with such an individual may be construed as preventing that person from obtaining medical services for the problem.

Make a medical referral (1) if the individual has a physical problem that seems to be getting worse instead of better or (2) if an acute sensitivity develops in any one of the stress cues. Without worrying the individual, ask whether he or she has seen a physician recently or suggest that he or she consult a physician.

Do not work on an undiagnosed problem   An undiagnosed problem is a problem that is acute enough to cause the client concern but which has not yet been examined by a physician. For example, a painful finger may be an injured finger that needs medical care. When in doubt, refer the client to medical personnel. Failure to refer to appropriate medical care is the chief concern of legal authorities about the services of complementary health practitioners.

The application of technique to a part of the foot or hand affected by a current injury is not appropriate. Consider the application of technique to the zone or referral area relevant to the foot or hand injury, although not directly on it. It may not even be possible to work on the foot or hand if the injury is such that you cannot hold the foot or apply technique within the comfort range of the individual. If the injury is serious and no medical services have been sought by the individual, refer the individual to a physician.

Do not work on an injured part of the foot

Confidentiality Code

It is the responsibility of the reflexologist to respect the client's privacy. Conversations between client and reflexologist should be held in strictest confidence. Observations made during work are to be held as confidential. Case study discussions are allowable among professionals but anonymity of the client must be maintained.

The Health Insurance Portability and Accountability Act (HIPAA) of 1996 requires, among other things, confidentiality. of health care services. Especially when insurance reimbursement is involved, the disclosure of any information about a client is limited to those (1) present at the session and, thus, considered to receive information with the client's permission or (2) who have been named by the client in a H. I. P. A. form.

The Workplace Environment

The reflexologist's office provides the tools of the trade for his or her work. Efficiency, comfort, and professionalism are considerations for the workplace. The reflexologist reflects his or her professionalism by what is available to the client to observe and to read in the workplace.
Both you and the individual should be comfortable during your reflexology work.

A recliner for the client and a low chair with back support for you help place the feet in a convenient and comfortable working position. To note the working position, drop your arms to your sides. Raise your hands, bending your elbow at approximately a 90° angle. A recliner also creates a working situation that allows you to maintain eye contact and watch the individual's reaction to your work. A throw pillow may be placed under the foot to raise it to a more convenient working position. If at all possible, work on bare feet. Nylons or stockings get in the way and are hard on the walking fingers.

Working position

Supplies   Handy supplies for the workplace include tissues, moistened towelettes, baby powder or corn starch, and bandages. Towelettes are made available for the convenience of the individual who wants to clean hot, sweaty, or dirty feet. Powder is utilized to dry a moist foot. Bandages are given to the individual to cover any open cut, thus protecting the area from technique application. A clock placed discreetly for your reference keeps your sessions on time. Pillows are useful to raise the foot if necessary to place it in position convenient for your work.

Cleanliness   The workplace should meet basic standards of sanitation. Facilities should be available to the client. who would like to wash his or her feet. Making moist towelettes available to the client is also a solution.

Products, books,
and charts   The reflexologist is responsible for anything in his or her workplace that can be read or handled by the client. Anything that gives the appearance of medical practice should be carefully considered. Any chart or book should contain a disclaimer noting that the information is not intended as a substitute for medical care.

Unless you are licensed to practice medicine, do not display or offer for sale in the workplace any herbs, vitamins, or ingestible products. Any product for sale or on display should fall within the standards and practices of the field of reflexology.

Business Ethics

Be ethical in all your dealings. Professional business practices are necessary to protect you and your reputation and that of reflexology as well. You should always be straightforward about fees, scheduling procedures, hours, and other information that could prevent misunderstandings later on.

Full and fair disclosure   To provide the consumer with the information he or she needs to make an intelligent choice in purchasing services, the reflexologist makes a full and fair disclosure of relevant information. The reflexologist provides specific information about his or her services: what the client is purchasing, how much it costs, what he or she can expect, and the reflexology credentials of the reflexologist.

Informed consent   A written statement, signed by the client, is a technique utilized to clearly signal that the purchaser of services has been fully and fairly informed about your services. An informed consent statement does not protect the reflexologist who is indeed practicing medicine without a license.

Do not advertise your reflexology business as a medical service. Listing specific ills can be hazardous to the health of any reflexology business. Business cards, "Yellow Pages" listings, promotional literature, and any other written material should not mention specific disorders.

Advertising

Certificates noting reflexology education and membership in professional organizations as well as a posted code of ethics provide professional credentials and an indication of full and fair disclosure of services.

Posting professional credentials

To clearly indicate the nature of reflexology services, the reflexologist talks in terms of reflexology, using the vocabulary of the field. Expertise in the profession is signaled by verbally conveying knowledge of the field and its terminology. Use of vocabulary from other professions serves to confuse the consumer about what service is being provided. (See "Professional Boundaries.") Terms such as cure, heal, therapy, treatment, massage, and manipulate signal the vocabulary of professions and bodies of knowledge other than reflexology.

Vocabulary use

The Working Reflexologist

Safety Issues

Before commencing work, briefly inspect the client's feet for cuts, rashes or injuries. Avoid cuts or injuries by placing a bandage over the area to make the session as safe as possible. Ask the client if any part of the foot should be avoided.

The visual inspection

Washing your hands before and between sessions is a necessity. It assures the client of cleanliness and a professional approach in the prevention of communicable disease.

Washing your hands

Communicable diseases are spread through the ingestion (eating or drinking) or inhalation (breathing) of bacteria or virus organisms or their toxins. This may occur either directly or indirectly. Many disease-causing organisms are commonly found in the intestinal tract, oral cavity, and nose of both ill and healthy persons. Illness occurs when these organisms are transferred to other persons or when they are transferred to another site in the body. Examples of direct transmission include instances in which an infected person (carrier) coughs or spits and airborne organisms are the inhaled by nearby persons, or when an infected person fails to wash the hands following urination or defecation and organisms are transmitted by touching another individual and that person ingests the organisms. Direct transmissions may also occur when organisms are transferred from an infected skin lesion or dirty hands to an open cut in the skin.

According to public health professionals, hand washing, when done correctly, is one of the most effective ways of preventing the spread of communicable diseases. Good hand washing technique is easy to learn and can significantly reduce the spread of infectious diseases in both children and adults.

Hands should be thoroughly washed following coughing, sneezing, rubbing the nose or defecation. Proper hand washing can effectively reduce the incidence of illnesses such as staphylococcus infections, salmonellas, typhoid fever, influenza, and the common cold. It should be noted that this is effective in reducing illness for both the reflexologists and client.

How to wash your hands

There is more to hand washing than you think. By rubbing your hands vigorously with soapy water, you pull the dirt plus the oily soils free from your skin. The soap lather suspends both the dirt and germs trapped inside and are then quickly washed away.

Follow these four simple steps to keeping hands clean:
• Wet your hands with warm running water.
• Add soap, then rub your hands together, making a soapy lather. Do this away from the running water for at least 10 seconds, being careful not to wash the lather away. Wash the front and back of your hands, as well as between your fingers and under your nails.
• Rinse your hands well under warm running water. Let the water run back into the sink, not down to your elbows. Turn off the sink with a paper towel and dispose in a proper receptacle.
• Dry hands thoroughly with a clean towel.

Type of soap

Any type of soap may be used. However, bar soap should be kept in a self draining holder that is cleaned thoroughly before new bars are put out and liquid soap containers (which must be used in day care centers) should be used until empty and cleaned before refilling. To prevent chapping use a mild soap with warm water, pat rather than rub hands dry, and apply lotion liberally and frequently.

Hand washing don't's

• DON'T use a standing basin of water to rinse hands.
• DON'T use a common hand towel. Always use disposable towels.
• DON'T use sponges or non-disposable cleaning cloths unless you launder them on a regular basis, adding chlorine bleach to the wash water. Remember that germs thrive on moist surfaces!

Research has shown that there is no potential for the spread of AIDS through skin contact. There is a problem, however, with blood to blood contact, exposure of an open wound to an open wound on another individual. There is a general rule of thumb for reflexologists: any breach in the skin is covered with a bandage and is to be avoided. The reflexologist should be aware of any breaches in his or her skin that could become exposed.

AIDS concerns

Use a common sense approach to such concerns. Keep bandages in your workplace so that you can provide one to any client to cover any open wound on his or her foot. Carefully consider your own work if you have an open cut or rash on your own hands.

Technique Application

Basic guidelines for technique application ensure the safety and comfort of your client. Consideration of how and where to apply technique provide is a part of the reflexologist's professional role.

The nails of the reflexologist's walking finger and thumb should not make contact with the skin of the foot at any time. Keep in mind, however, that it is possible for fingernails to be too short. The nail will pull away from the skin and can cause pain. Take the time to check your fingernail length and cleanliness at the beginning of work everyday. Keep nail files or clippers handy to maintain an appropriate length.

Fingernail length

The client's comfort level is the primary determinant of the amount of pressure to be exerted. Tastes vary from client to client. To establish an individual client's preference, ask the client to indicate discomfort due to the pressure exerted. Some clients may even request additional pressure. The goal of the practitioner is to stay within the client's comfort zone.

Maintain a comfort level

Pain is not an activity that needs to be practiced. There is a difference between a client's comment of, "It hurts good" and one of "It hurts." One method of eliciting comments on the amount of pressure preferred by the client is to ask, "Will you tell me if the pressure is too much?" This is an especially appropriate question when applying techniques to areas you think might be sensitive; for example, working with the pancreas reiterative area of a diabetic.

Respect an individual's response to pain

A thirty to forty-five minute session is considered to be an appropriate length of time for technique application. A session that lasts more than an hour can overtax the client and create a reaction – flulike symptoms or discomfort caused by the release of toxins or waste products in the system.

Duration of a foot reflexology session

Shorter session are applied with children. Shorter, more frequent sessions are utilized with the ill. A full-length session may overtax an already taxed body.

Instruments and tools

In reflexology, instruments are utilized as self-help tools. Instruments have no ability to feel and thus have no place in a reflexologist's practice. The easiest way to pursue safe, effective techniques is with hands on technique application.

Creams, lotions and goo

Creams, lotions, and oils are tools of foot massage. While foot massage is a valid practice in itself, it is not the same as foot reflexology. The techniques of reflexology require friction between the walking thumb and the skin of the hand. Use of creams, lotions, and oils at the end of a session is an individual practitioner decision. Note, however, that the practitioner's hands become covered with the cream, lotion or oil and their presence will be a factor in the session with the following client.

Reactions

Occasionally after a session an individual may have a disagreeable reaction. Normally this will be a feeling of general discomfort or flu-like symptoms. Do not panic if this happens. Reassure your client by explaining that this is common and should pass quickly. If the problem does seem to continue, however, it may not be a reaction to the session and you should suggest that your client seek medical help.

Analyze your approach if disagreeable reactions are a regular occurrence. Perhaps you are not emphasizing work on the reflex areas for kidney, bladder, lymph, intestinal, and other organs of elimination, especially during the first few sessions with an individual. Also, you may be working too long or too much. Remember that reflexology is a conditioning process. Just as with any exercise program, start your work gradually, build up, and don't overdo.

If the individual has a disagreeable reaction during your work, back away from pressure technique application and go to desserts. Stop altogether if the reaction continues. Consider your work to be overtaxing to the individual at this time.

Foot baths and massage machines

The use of foot baths and massage machines with reflexology services should be carefully considered for safety reasons. Questions about cleanliness have created an issue about the use of foot baths in professional services. No standards exist to gauge the service of machine-applied technique.

Self-help is the involvement of the client in his or her own program of wellness. Reflexology provides technique application that is an opportunity to practice and exercise the foot's capabilities. The addition of the client's self-help program is an opportunity to spend more time exercising. (For information about self-help reflexology techniques, see *Reflexology, Health at your fingertips,* Barbara and Kevin Kunz, DK, 2003 or *Hand and Foot Reflexology, A Self-Help Guide,* Barbara and Kevin Kunz, Simon and Schuster, 1984.)

The role of the reflexologist as an advocate of self-help

The Business of Reflexology

When considering the business of reflexology, consider the potential for income and expense. If you're launching your own practice, there will be both business and workplace expenses. If you're working for another, you'll be splitting your fees with the proprietor of the establishment. The bottom line is your bottom line. If you are new to the business world, classes in small business start-up and operation are available.

Consider also expanding your reflexology business by expanding your reflexology education and services. Gaining skills in self-help reflexology and hand reflexology enables you to provide these services. Consider also whether or not receiving insurance payments is appropriate for your business. (See "Insurance Reimbursement for Reflexology Services.")

Income

First, how much will you charge for your reflexology services? Fees for reflexology services vary from one region of the country to another ranging from $35 to $200 per session. In setting your fee, consider what the market will bear - what do others charge? Consider how many client sessions will be required per week to meet your expenses and living wage. In addition, consider how much time will be required to build your business up to the point you're seeing this number of clients. Reports of success from satisfied clients are the backbone of any reflexology practice. Many reflexologists build their businesses by working part time, first achieving results with family and friends and a limited clientele. With the establishment of word-of-mouth success stories, the reflexologist goes on to a fuller practice.

Expenses

Calculating expense is a part of any business. You'll want to consider the costs of setting up your both a business and a reflexology workplace

Workplace expenses include cost of the your location and the reflexologist's basic equipment.

Business expenses

Business expenses include business cards, telephone, telephone book listing, brochures, and advertising. A "Reflexologist" listing in the Yellow Pages is available in many regions. Telephone books are printed once a year. Check to see when your listing will enter the cycle. Aside from a business listing in white pages and Yellow Pages, advertising is available.

The mobile reflexologist

Some reflexologists have by-passed the expense of an office location by becoming mobile. The mobile reflexologist pays visits to clients' homes or workplaces. Expenses are minimal: a portable reclining chair for the client and a working chair for the reflexologist. On the other hand, while the overhead of an office is avoided, more time is required to move from location to location. Transportation is needed as well. In addition, working in someone's home or office will involve you more in their family and work life. Aside from involving your time, you'll be stepping into the client's relationships. You'll find yourself petting dogs and getting to know family members or office mates.

The reflexology workplace

Renting office space is an expense to be carefully considered. Location, cost and appropriateness to your business are primary considerations. An easy-to-reach location with adequate parking and handicap accessibility are important. Price range, cleanliness and rest room availability are also important. A waiting room and session room are minimal. Sharing office space is a possibility. Consider compatibility with both the potential office mate and his or her business.

Ambiance is the next consideration. You can add decor elements such as art, fountains or a music system to create a more pleasant environment for your client's experience.

Working for another

Typically, working for another includes splitting the reflexologist's fee with the proprietor of the business. Before entering into any arrangement consider the business terms and relationship: what is the fee split, when are monies paid to you, how many client referrals can be expected, and what are the workplace conditions. Has reflexology been offered at the business previously?

Answering queries

When a prospective client calls, be prepared to cite your fees, location and recite your training and experience. Be familiar with reflexology research. When asked, Can you help me with _____ (a specific disorder), be knowledgeable and state, Research has shown effectiveness or Yes, I have worked with that before. (Indicating that you treat for a specific disorder is counter to professional ethics and potentially the medical practices act.)

Insurance Reimbursement for Reflexology Services

"Do you take insurance?" It's a question commonly asked of reflexologists by potential clients. The answer is, yes, insurance reimbursement for reflexology services is available - under certain circumstances.

If you've ever had a visit to a doctor paid by an insurance company, you've encountered a key component for payment in the medical industry ... coding. If you see a doctor for a sore throat, for example, the doctor's office goes to a coding book, finds the code appropriate for the sore throat treatment and bills the insurance company using that number. Coding for reflexology services is available. In addition to making reimbursement possible, coding makes it possible to track the effectiveness of reflexology.

The reflexologist, client, and the client's insurance company must meet specifications. The reflexologist must be able to provide proof of educational and credentialing qualifications to the insurance company. The reflexologist must be covered by malpractice insurance. The client's employer must provide health insurance that includes coverage for complementary and integrative practices. Next, the client must be included in such a program. The program must include reflexology services. Not all programs include reflexology services. Some programs, however, include discretionary accounts, i. e. flexible medical spending accounts, that allow the individual to choose services such as reflexology.

The insurance company may not authorize reimbursement for reflexology services. It may be easiest to ask the client to pay and then submit a claim with the insurance company themselves.

Reflexologists are allowed to provide certain precise interventions for which they are qualified: foot reflexology, hand reflexology and reflexology assessment. Filing a claim and accepting payment outside of allowed procedures can result in charges of insurance fraud, punishable by up to $10,000 in fines per line item.

How to start

Paperwork for insurance reimbursement includes filing a Standard Claims Form with the insurance company. A "Reflexology Super Bill" that includes necessary information is available through at www.foot-reflexologist.com. Purchase of a coding book is suggested to become educated and aware of the possibilities as well as to keep on hand as a reference when filing the Super Bill. An additional resource is the *ABC Coding Manual for*

Integrative Healthcare listing all interventions allowed by qualified providers of complementary and integrated therapies available at www.foot-reflexologist.com.

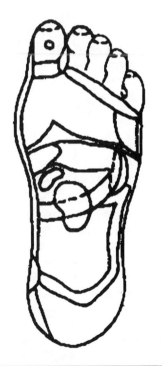

6

Reflexology Research

The role of research in the reflexologist's professional life is to: (1) add to one's credibility with clientele and other health professionals; (2) contribute to the one's confidence with the realization of the potential impact of the practice and one's work on the health of others; (3) frame reflexology's effectiveness in a proper manner; and (4) understand how and why reflexology works.

To put reflexology research into its proper perspective, several facts emerge. There is an abundance of research of a high quality. Most of it shows a positive impact of reflexology work. Research is on-going. It is also largely ignored until and unless the reflexologist makes it known.

This chapter details research fundamentals as well as specific reflexology research. Such knowledge provides you with credible information to communicate to clients and other professionals. Use of research facts allows you to speak to the effectiveness of reflexology work applied to those with specific disorders without making claims. In addition, research information leads to your growth as a reflexologist, providing a focus for your work and an ability to problem solve based on a logical understanding of what reflexology does and does not do.

Research Basics

When reflexology (or any drug or therapy) is considered for use by the medical community, specific criteria are considered. These standards are utilized to determine (1) whether or not the therapy is useful in treating a specific disorder, (2) whether or not it is more useful than other procedures, and (3) whether or not it works better than a placebo, an inactive pill or procedure. During research, a therapy or drug is tested for its:

Safety: Safety of approach is a matter of concern within the medical community. Research provides to the medical community evidence that an approach will do no harm and that it is safer than other therapies.

Cost-effectiveness: Cost is a factor in choosing among treatment options. At issue is whether one treatment is less costly but as effective as another.

Efficacy: The efficacy or effectiveness of an approach is a primary concern in research. In medical research, specific phrases signify level of efficacy: significantly effective, effective and no effect.

Mechanism of Action: A mechanism of action describes how or why a therapy or drug achieves results. Some studies are conducted simply to test the mechanism at work.

Research Quality

The quality of research is judged by its approach. Some studies are given more credibility than others. As you read through the following, keep in mind that double-blind, randomized controlled studies have the most validity.

Survey: "A survey is a kind of study that reports the results of interviewing people....

Clinical trial: "A clinical trial is one in which the subjects are human....

Case study: "A case study is a report on one unusual subject by a doctor. ... a case series should consist of at least five cases....

Randomized study: "A randomized trial is one in which subjects are assigned to different groups as randomly as possible - by flipping a coin or a random number generator. ...

Controlled study: "In a controlled trial at least two groups are compared. The treated or experimental group receives the intervention, while the other - called the control group - or simply the control - doesn't. Or different groups may receive different interventions....

Single-blind technique: "In a single blind study, the subjects don't know (whether they are in the treatment group or control group) but the researchers do..."[1]

"Double-blinded technique: A method of scientific investigation in which neither the subject not the investigator working with the subject or analyzing the data knows what treatment, if any, the subject is receiving. At the completion of the experiment, the 'code' is broken and data are analyzed with respect to the various treatments used. This method completely eliminates any bias by the observer or subject."[2]

Research into Specific Disorders

Both prospective clientele and medical personnel have an interest in information about research and reflexology's ability to impact a specific disorder. Clientele have an interest because such information provides a type of buyer's assurance that reflexology has credibility. For medical personnel, such research meets a basic criteria of proof for use of a treatment within scientific parameters - the therapy has been found to be safe and effective.

[1.] Fuch-Berman, Adriane, *Alternative Medicine: What Works*, "Scientific Terms Explained," Odonian Press, Tucson, Arizona, 1996, p. 11

[2.] *Taber's Cyclopedic Medical Dictionary*, F. A. Davis Co., Philadelphia, 1981, p. 427

A question frequently asked by a prospective client is, Can you help me with _____ (a specific health problem)? The knowledge that a study about the effectiveness of reflexology has been conducted on those with the disorder provides a credible answer to the individual without making a claim. Case in point: The telephone rings and a prospective client says, Can you help me with diabetes? An appropriate answer would be: There have been studies showing the impact of reflexology on diabetes as well as improved blood flow to the feet of diabetics.

Controlled Studies by System

The following brief descriptions of studies can be utilized to describe the benefits of reflexology. These studies were selected because they are all controlled studies. The studies are grouped by the body's systems. Diabetes, for example, is a disorder of the endocrine system and studies would thus be listed under "Endocrine System." The purpose of grouping by the body's systems is to allow generalization. While not each and every disorder has been studied, there may be a similar effect among disorders of a system.

Not all of the following studies showed a positive impact of reflexology on a disorder. When discussing a study with a negative outcome, be honest. Instead of surmising that reflexology is a cure-all, try to objectify the information as would any professional.

The numbers following the brief descriptions cite the published source of the research, found in the "Bibliography of Controlled Studies" at the end of this chapter. A fuller description of each study can be found at www.reflexology-research.com.

Cancer / Hospice

• Reflexology work reduced pain and nausea in patients hospitalized with cancer. (2c)
• Reflexology work improved quality of life for palliative patients. (2d)
• Foot reflexology alleviated anxiety and pain for twenty-three patients with breast and lung cancer. (2e)
• Hand massage reduced nausea, vomiting, anxiety in children undergoing chemotherapy. (2f)
• Foot reflexology significantly decreased nausea, vomiting, and fatigue of breast cancer patients undergoing chemotherapy. (2g)

Cardio-Vascular System

• Individuals who receive foot reflexology showed an improvement in symptoms of hyperlipimia (cholesterol and monoglyceride). (16)

• Symptoms of coronary heart disease (chest distress and angina) disappeared in those receiving foot reflexology work as well as causing a drop in blood pressure of 25/5, results better than those achieved with medication.(9)

• "The reflexology and foot massage control groups experienced a significantly greater reduction in baroreceptor reflex sensitivity,..." "the mechanism that maintains blood pressure and homeostasis by changes in autonomic outflow." (3)

Dermatology

• Foot reflexology was found to avoid the side effects of drug therapy such as fatigue, sleeplessness and gastrointestinal symptoms in treating neurodermatitis. (22)

Digestive System

• Not only did constipated individuals evacuate their bowels more quickly when receiving reflexology work but individuals with normal bowel function do also. (8)

• Foot reflexology work was found to be more effective than drugs in treating dyspepsia. (13)

• Reflexology work did not influence irritable bowel syndrome. (17b)

Endocrine System

• Diabetic individuals provided with foot reflexology and hypoglycemic agents showed a significant change in measures of the disease as opposed to those who received hypoglycemic agents alone where no significant change was observed. (10)

• For individuals diagnosed as diabetic, hypoglycemic agents worked better for those receiving reflexology work as well as showing "marked improvement" in measures of the disease. (11)

• There were significant differences in the blood flow rate to the feet of Type II diabetes individuals before and after application of technique. (12)

Gerontology

• The self-help reflexology technique of walking on a cobblestone mat was found to lessen blood pressure and pain as well as increase a sense of control over falls in senior citizens.

Immune System

• Foot reflexology work was found to be more effective than medication in effecting leukopenia, low white blood cell count. (19)

Mental Health
• Alzheimer's patients saw a reduction in body stiffness and arthritis as well as alleviation of the illness's symptoms of restlessness and wandering. (1)

Musculo-Skeletal System
• Individuals with cervical spondylosis were found to experience a higher clinical cure rate than those treated with traction. (5)

Nervous System
• 19% of headache sufferers ceased taking medication following reflexology work. (15)
• For individuals suffering from migraine headache, reflexology treatment was at least as effective as the Flunarizin treatment and may be classified as an alternative non-pharmacological therapeutic treatment that would be particularly appropriate to those patients that were unable to follow pharmacological treatment." (15a)
• Symptoms of those with multiple sclerosis improved following foot reflexology work. (19d)
• Specific reflexology treatment was of benefit in alleviating motor; sensory and urinary symptoms in multiple sclerosis patients. 19e)

Pediatrics
• Children with cerebral palsy who received reflexology work showed an improved growth rate over those who did not. (4)
• Mentally retarded children were shown to improve significantly in height, weight, health states, social living abilities, and intellectual development when receiving foot reflexology as opposed to those not receiving treatment. (7)
• The feet of mentally retarded children were found to be of abnormal color and show abnormal shapes in toes as opposed to other children. (6)
• Infants who received both medication and reflexology work recovered from infantile pneumonia more quickly than those who received medication alone. (17)
• Reflexology work did not reduce the incidence of enuresis (bed wetting). (13b)

Post-surgical
• Post surgical patients who received foot massage and medication reported "significantly less" agony than those on painkillers alone. (23)
• Foot reflexology work with acute abdominal post surgical patients triggered pain. (23a)
• Post surgical women voided earlier following foot reflexology work but slept better and had less pain with foot massage.(23b)

Reproductive System

• Women who have recently given birth lactated earlier and more satisfactorily when given foot reflexology work. (21)

• 95% of women who experienced amenorrhea find foot reflexology to be effective. (2)

• Reflexology improved the symptoms of 46% of those suffering from PMS. (24)

• Reflexology was found to be 87.5% effective for men experiencing impotence and 100% effective for other male sexual dysfunctions. (26)

• Reflexology work did not reduce edema in pregnant women. (13a)

• Foot massage, but not hand massage, can evoke fetal activity in mid-gestat ion (13d)

• Foot reflexology was not found to impact symptoms of menopause. (Nine sessions over 19 weeks) (19b)

• Foot reflexology was found to impact symptoms of menopause. (Sixty sessions over 60 days) (19c)

Respiratory System

• There is no evidence that reflexology has a specific effect on asthma beyond a placebo influence. (2a) (2b)

Skeletal System

• Reflexology work was not found to impact low back pain. (19a)

Urinary System

• Individuals who received lithotrity (external mechanical impact on kidney or ureter stones) expelled the fragmented stones more quickly with foot reflexology work. (28)

• Reflexology work reduced the pain of those with kidney and ureter stones. (20)

• Lithotrity (external crushing of kidney and ureter stones) patients experienced less pain, began excretion of stones earlier, and completed excretion earlier than those who did not receive reflexology work. (18)

• Reflexology work was found to be more effective and safer than the standard treatment of catheterization in patients with uroschesis, retention of urine following surgery. (30)

• Individuals with kidney infection who received foot reflexology and medication recovered more quickly than those who used medicine alone. (29)

Mechanisms and Techniques

• Foot reflexology work was found to decrease the free radicals present in test subjects. (14)

• Reflexology work resulted in improved blood flow to the intestines. (17a)

• Reflexology work applied to the kidney reflex area was found to improve blood flow to and influence function of the kidneys. (18a)

Miscellaneous
• Reflexology reduced the pain of 66% toothache patients as well eliminating the symptoms of 26%. (27)
• Reflexology saved one Danish employer US$3, 300 a month in fewer sick days for employees in addition to improving the work environment. (31)
• Reflexology reduced fatigue in athletes. (13c)
• "Reflexology massage" was found to be as effective as nasal irrigation for alleviation of chronic sinusitis. (26a)

Criteria for Medical Applications

It is the role of research to aid medical personnel in determining the potential application of therapies to consumers of medical services. Medical personnel are interested to know that reflexology has been shown scientifically to have an impact on the body. Two types of research provide such information. As noted previously, research applied to those with a specific disorder can show that reflexology work is not only effective but also safe. Another type of research tests for a mechanism of action.

A mechanism of action describes how or why a therapy or drug achieves results. Such a study is of value to the reflexologist for several reasons. One, it shows that reflexology is proven to physically impact the body. Two, such studies show the possibility of an over-lying principle causing impact in a variety of disorders.

Reflexology Mechanism of Action

For the professional reflexologist, an ability to discuss how reflexology works creates value in the service being purchased by a client or considered by medical personnel. In other words, credibility and legitimacy for a reflexology service are created by a practitioner who can describe in specific terms what takes place as reflexology technique is applied to the feet or hands.

There is no universal agreement about the mechanism involved in reflexology work. Several theories could apply. For example, 36 of 153 Chinese studies surveyed included a discussion of mechanisms. Two significant observations emerge from these: (1) all view multiple mechanisms at work in reflexology technique application and (2) all view at least one of the mechanisms to be within the nervous system. Improved blood circulation is most frequently mentioned. Frequently mentioned also is improved function through what might be considered an exercise effect — a stimulation and response of the nervous system to condition a better regulation of the body.

Two Austrian studies support improved blood circulation as a mechanism of action. One study showed that reflexology influences blood flow to the kidneys (18a) and the other demonstrated an influence on blood flow to the intestines (18b). Both were randomized, controlled double-blind studies that measured blood flow with a Doppler sonogram before and after reflexology work.

Among mechanisms used to describe the effect of reflexology the following are most commonly cited:
• **Endorphin release:** Pain-killing endorphins are released when the pain threshold is altered in response to technique application.
• **Circulation:** Lymphatic and blood circulation is improved through physical application of technique.
• **Nerve supply:** Technique application provides nerve stimulation that prompts the nerves to work better.
• **Nervous system:** Technique application provides sensory (afferent) nervous system input that influences (efferent) autonomic and motor nervous system output.
• **Impact on anti-oxidation**: Technique application stimulates nerve fibers bringing about a change in physiological responses specifically improving the systemic blood circulation and metabolism, decreasing the production of free radicals, increasing the production of antioxidative enzymes and achieving the therapeutic effect.
• **Psychological benefit:** The client benefits from interaction with caring, listening practitioner.
• **Energy balance:** Benefits result from a balance of qi or chi, an energy system of the body outside of the nervous system.
• **Relaxation:** A physiological reduction in stress results from technique application.
• **Placebo:** Reflexology results in a placebo effect defined as an inactive pill or procedure that makes one feel better for no apparent reason.

Bibliography of Controlled Studies

1. Alzheimer's "Old age converts to the New Age," *Daily Mail*, September 14, 1995

2. Amenorrhea Xiu-hua, Xu, "Analysis of 50 Cases of Amenorrhea Treated by Foot Reflex Therapy," *(19)96 Beijing International Reflexology Conference (Report),* China Preventive Medical Association and the Chinese Society of Reflexology, Beijing, 1996, p. 36

2a. Asthma Brygge T, Heinig JH, Collins P, Ronborg SM, Gehrchen PM, Hilden J, Heegaard S, Poulsen LK, "Zone Therapy and Asthma," Ugeskr Laeger, 2002, Apr. 29; 164(18):2405-10 (Danish language)

2b. Petersen LN, Faurschou P, Olsen OT, Svendsen UG. Ugeskr Laeger. 1992 Jul 20;154(30):2065-8. Ugeskr Laeger. 1993 Feb 1;155(5):329-31. Lungemedicinsk/allergologisk afdeling Y, Kobenhavns Amts Sygehus i Gentofte

Cancer (pain and nausea, quality of life)

2c. Grealish, L. Lomasney, A., Whiteman, B., "Foot Massage: A nursing intervention to modify the distressing symptoms of pain and nausea in patients hospitalized with cancer," *Cancer Nurse 2000*, June;23(3):237-43 (On-line review: "Reflexology Used for Cancer Patients," Internet Health Library, October 11, 2000)

2d. Hodgson, H. "Does reflexology impact on cancer patients' quality of life?," *Nursing Standard*, 14, 31, pp. 33-38

2e. Stephenson, N. L., Weinrich, S. P. and Tavakoli, A. S., "The effects of foot reflexology on anxiety and pain in patients with breast and lung cancer," *OncolNursForum 2000*, Jan.-Feb.;27(1):67-72

2f. Ji-Eun Han, Master, RN, Young-Im Moon, Ph.D., and Ho-Ran Park, Ph.D. "Effect of Hand Massage on Nausea, Vomiting and Anxiety of Childhood Acute Lymphocytic Leukemia with High Dose Chemotherapy," Presented at Back to Evidence-Based Nursing: Strategies for Improving Practice, Sigma Theta Tau International, July 21, 2004

2g. Yang, JH, "The effects of foot reflexology on nausea, vomiting and fatigue of breast cancer patients undergoing chemotherapy" Taechan Kanho Hakhoe Chie, 2005 Feb;35(1):177-85

3. Cardio-vascular system Frankel, B. S. M., "The effect of reflexology on baroreceptor reflex sensitivity, blood pressure and sinus arrhythmia," *Complementary Therapies in Medicine*, Churchill, London, 1997, Vol. 5, pp. 80-84

4. Cerebral palsy Rong-zhi, Wang, "An Approach to Treatment of Cerebral Palsy of Children by Foot Massage," A Clinical Analysis of 132 Cases," *(19)96 Beijing International Reflexology Conference (Report),* China Preventive Medical Association and the Chinese Society of Reflexology, Beijing, 1996, p. 26

5. Cervical spondylosis Shouqing, Gui; Changlong, Zhang and Desheng, Luo, "A Controlled Clinical Observation on Foot Reflexology Treatment for Cervical Spondylopathy,"*1996 China Reflexology Symposium Report*, China Reflexology Association, Beijing, pp. 99-103

6. Children, mentally retarded, Feng, Gu; Zhao, Lingyun; Yuru, Yang; Jiamo, Hao; Shuwen, Cao and Xiulan, Zhang, "Comparative Study of Abnormal Signs in the Feet of Feebleminded Children, *1998China Reflexology Symposium Report*, China Reflexology Association, Beijing, pp. 9 - 13

7. Lingyun, Yuru, Zhao; Yang Yuru, Feng gu; Jiamo, Hao; Shuwen, Cao and Xiulan, Zhang, "Observation on Improvement of Feeble-Minded Children's Social Abilities by Foot Reflexo-Therapy," *1998 China Reflexology Symposium Report*, China Reflexology Association, Beijing, pp. 24 - 28

8. Constipation Yuru, Yang; Lingyun, Chao; Guangling, Meng; Scuwe, Cao; Jia-Mo, Hao and Suhui, Zhang, "Exploring the Application of Foot Reflexology to the Preventions and Treatment of Functional Constipation," *1994 China Reflexology Symposium Report*, China Reflexology Association, Beijing, p. 62

9. Coronary heart disease Zhongzheng, Li and Yuchun, Liu, "Clinical observation on Treatment of Coronary Heart Disease with Foot Reflexotherapy, *1998 China Reflexology Symposium Report*, China Reflexology Association, Beijing, pp. 38 - 41

10. Diabetes Wang, X. M., "Type II diabetes mellitus with foot reflexotherapy," *Chuang Koh Chuang Hsi I Chief Ho Teas Chi,* Beijing, Vol. 13, Sept. 1993, pp 536-538

11. Zhi-qin, Duan et. al., "Foot Reflexology Therapy Applied On Patients with NIDDM (non-insulin dependent diabetic mellitus)," *1993 China Reflexology Symposium*, p. 24

12. King, Ma, "Clinical Observation on Influence upon Arterial Blood Flow in the Lower Limbs of 20 Cases with Type II Diabetes Mellitus Treated by Foot Reflexology," *1998 China Reflexology Symposium Report*, CRA, Beijing, pp. 97 - 99

12a. Diagnosis White, AR, Williamson, J. and Ernst, E., "Foot Reflexology: A Sole Method of Diagnosis?, *Fact: Focus on Alternative and Complementary Therapies 1998;* 3(4) (Report from the Fifth Annual Symposium on Complementary Health Care, University of Exeter)

13. Dyspepsia Zhi-wen, Gong and Wei-song, Xin, "Foot Reflexology in the Treatment of Functional Dyspepsia: A Clinical Analysis of 132 Cases," *(19)96 Beijing International Reflexology Conference (Report),* China Preventive Medical Association and the Chinese Society of Reflexology, Beijing, 1996, p. 37

13a. Edema Mollart l., "Single Blind trial addressing the differential effects of two reflexology techniques versus rest, on ankle and foot oedema in late pregnancy," *Complement Ther Nurs Midwifery,* 2003 Nov;9(4):203-8)

13b. Comment in: Ugeskr Laeger 1999 Apr 12;161(15):2224 Sietam KS, Eriksen L Forenede Danske Zoneterapeuter, Kolding.

13 c. Fatigue Jianguo, Liu and Jingshun, Zhang, "Foot Reflex Zone Massage in Recovery of Fatigue in Athletes," *1994 China Reflexology Symposium Report,* China Reflexology Association, Beijing, p. 98

13d. Fetal activity Diego MA, Dieter JN, Field T, Lecanuet JP, Hernandez-Reif M, Beutler J, Largie S, Redzepi M, Salman FA., "Fetal activity following stimulation of the mother's abdomen, feet, and hands," *Dev Psychobiol.* 2002 Dec;41(4):396-406

14. Free radicals Shouqing, Gui; Changlong, Zhang; Jixai, Dong and Desheng, Luoof, "A Preliminary Study on the Mechanisms of Foot Reflexo-Massage — Its Effect on Free Radicals," *1996 China Reflexology Symposium Report,* China Reflexology Association, Beijing, pp. 128-135

Gerontology Fuzhong Li; Peter Harmer; Nicole L. Wilson; K. John Fisher, "Health Benefits of Cobble-Stone Mat Walking: Preliminary Findings," Journal of Aging and Physical Activity, 11(4), October 2003

15. Headaches Brendstrup, Eva and Launsø, Laila, "Headache and Reflexological Treatment," The Council Concerning Alternative Treatment, The National Board of Health, Denmark, 1997; Launso, Laila, Brendstrup, Eva, and Arnberg, Soren, "An Exploration of Reflexological Treatment for Headache," Alternative Therapies, May 1999, Vol. 5, No. 3, pp. 57 - 65

15a Headache (Migraine) Testa, Gail W., "A Study on the Effects of Reflexology on Migraine Headaches" August 2000 (http://members.tripod.com/GTesta/Dissertationall.htm)

Lafuente A et al (1990). Effekt der Reflex zonenbehandlung am FuB bezuglich der prophylaktischen Behandlung mit Flunarizin bei an Cephalea-Kopfschmerzen leidenden Patieten.Erfahrungsheilkunde. 39, 713-715.

16. Hyperlipimia Shou-qing, Gui; Xian-qing, Xiao; Yuna-zhong, Li; and Wan-yan, Fu, "Impact of the Massotherapy Applied to Foot Reflexes on Blood Fat of Human Body," *1996 China Reflexology Symposium Report,* China Reflexology Association, Beijing, p. 21

17. Infantile Pneumonia Liang-cai, Pei, "Observation of 58 Infantile Pneumonia by Combined Method of Medication with Foot Massage," A Clinical Analysis of 132 Cases," *(19)96 Beijing International Reflexology Conference (Report),* China Preventive Medical Association and the Chinese Society of Reflexology, Beijing, 1996, p. 34

17a. Intestines (Blood flow as a mechanism of action) J, Egger I, Bodner G, Eibl G, Hartig F, Pfeiffer KP, Herold M., "Influence of reflex zone therapy of the feet on intestinal blood flow measured by color Doppler sonography," [Article in German] Forsch Komplementarmed Klass Naturheilkd. 2001 Apr;8(2):86-9. (Universitatsklinik fur Innere Medizin, Innsbruck, Austria)

17b. Irritable bowel syndrome Dr. Phillip Tovey, Published in *British Journal of General Practice* (Reported December 31, 2001 at http://news.bbc.co.uk/hi/english/health/newsid_1723000/17232900.stm)

18. Kidney and Ureter Stones Xiaojian, Ying, "Foot Reflexology as an Accessory Treatment after External Lithotrity, *1996 China Reflexology Symposium Report,* China Reflexology Association, Beijing, p. 58 - 59

18a Kidney (blood flow to) Sudmeier, I., Bodner, G., Egger, I., Mur, E., Ulmer, H. and Herold, M. (Universitatsklinik fur Innere Medizin, Inssbruk, Austria) "Anderung der nierendurchblutung durch organassoziierte reflexzontherapie am fuss gemussen mit farbkodierter doppler-sonograhpie," *Forsch Komplementarmed* 1999, Jum;6(3):129-34 (PMID: 14060981, UI: 99392031)

19. Leukopenia (Pathological level of white blood cell count) Ya-zhen, Xu, "Treatment of Leukopenia with Reflexotherapy," *1998 China Reflexology Symposium Report,* China Reflexology Association, Beijing, pp. 32-7

19a. Low back pain Poole, H. M., Murphy, P., & Glenn, S. "Evaluating the efficacy of reflexology for chronic back pain," *The Journal of Pain*, 2(2), 47 (http://www.ampainsoc.org/abstract/2001/data/221/)

19b. Menopause Williamson J, White A, Hart A, Ernst E., Randomised controlled trial of reflexology for menopausal symptoms, BJOG, 2002 Sep; 109(9):1050-5 (PMID: 12269681)

19c. Menopause Sun Jianhua, "Observation on the Therapeutic Effect of 82 Cases of Climacterium Syndrome (menopause) Treated with Reflexotherapy," *1998 China Reflexology Symposium Report*, China Reflexology Association, Beijing, pp. 60-61

19d. Multiple sclerosis Joyce M, Richardson R. "Reflexology helps multiple sclerosis," *JACM* July 1997 10-12

19e. Multiple sclerosis Siev-Ner I, Gamus D, Lerner-Geva L, Achiron A., "Reflexology treatment relieves symptoms of multiple sclerosis: a randomized controlled study," *Mult Scler.* 2003 Aug;9(4):356-61

20. Pain of kidney and ureter stones Eriksen, Leila, "Clinical Trials of Acute Uretic Colic and Reflexology," *Reflexology: Research and Effect Evaluation in Denmark*, Danish Reflexologists Association, Kolding, Denmark, 1993, p. 10

21. Milk secretion in new mothers Siu-lan, Li, "Galactagogue Effect of Foot Reflexology in 217 Parturient Women," *(19)96 Beijing International Reflexology Conference (Report)*, China Preventive Medical Association and the Chinese Society of Reflexology, Beijing, 1996 p. 14

22. Neurodermatitis Zhi-ming, Liu and Song, Fang, "Treatment of Neurodermatitis by Foot Reflex Area Massage," *(19)96 Beijing International Reflexology Conference (Report)*, China Preventive Medical Association and the Chinese Society of Reflexology, Beijing, 1996, p. 16

23. Post surgical pain "Foot Rubs Easing Pain," Third Age. com, December 4, 1998

23a. Post surgical pain Kesselring A., "Foot Reflexology massage: a clinical study." *Forsch Komplementarmed* 1999 Feb; 6 Suppl 1:38-40

23b. Post surgical recovery Kesselring A., Spichiger E., Muller M, "Foot Reflexology: an intervention study, *Pflege* 1998, Aug; 11(4):213-8

24. Pre-menstrual syndrome Oleson, Terry and Flocco, William, "Randomized Controlled Study of Premenstrual Symptoms Treated with Ear, Hand, and Foot Reflexology," *Obstetrics and Gynecology*, 1993;82(6): 906-11

25. (Hyperplasia of the) Prostate Xiao-li, Chen, "Hyperplasia of Prostate Gland Treated by Foot Reflex Area Health Promoting Method (with a group of 90 study participants)," *1996 China Reflexology Symposium Report*, China Reflexology Association, Beijing, October 1996, pp. 32 - 33

26. (Male) Sexual dysfunction Jianhua, Sun, "The Comparison of Curative Effects Between Foot Reflexology and Chinese Traditional Medicine in Treating 37 Cases with Male's Sexual Dysfunction,"

"Foot Reflexology as an Accessory Treatment after External Lithotrity a Clinical Observation of 46 Cases, *1996 China Reflexology Symposium Report*, China Reflexology Association, Beijing, p. 75

26a. Sinusitis Diane G. Heatley MD, Glen E. Leverson Ph.D., Kari E. McConnell RN, and Tony L. Kille, "Nasal Irrigation for the Alleviation of Sinonasal Symptoms," *Otolaryngol Head Neck Surg.* 2001 Jul;125(1):44-8)

27. Toothache Xue-xiang, Wang, "Relieve (150 Cases of) Toothache with Foot Reflexotherapy," *1994 China Reflexology Symposium Report*, China Reflexology Association, Beijing, October 1994, pp. 132 - 135

28. Urinary tract stones Yue-jin, Zhang; Jing-Fang, Chung and Bao-rong, Ju, "Observation of the Effect of Foot Reflex Area Massage on 34 Cases of Calouli of Urinary Tract," *(19)96 Beijing International Reflexology Conference (Report)*, *1996*, China Preventive Medical Association and the Chinese Society of Reflexology, Beijing, 1996, p. 46

29. Urinary tract infection Yu-lian, Zao, "Clinical Observation on Treatment of Infection of Urinary Tract by Foot Massage," *(19)96 Beijing International Reflexology Conference (Report)*, China Preventive Medical Association and the Chinese Society of Reflexology, Beijing, 1996, p. 17

30. Uroschesis (retention of urine) Cailian, Lin, "Clinical Observation on Treatment of 40 Cases of Uroschesis with Reflexology," *1998 China Reflexology Symposium Report*, China Reflexology Association, Beijing, pp. 52 - 53

31. Employee sick days Eriksen, Leila, *Reflexology: Research and Effect Evaluation in Denmark*, Danish Reflexologists Association, Denmark, August 1995, pp. 15 - 16

32. Strength of stimulation Feng Jinqi and Fan Chunmei, A Concept of Strength of Stimulation in Reflexology," *1996 China Symposium Reflexology Report*, China Reflexology Association, Beijing, 1996

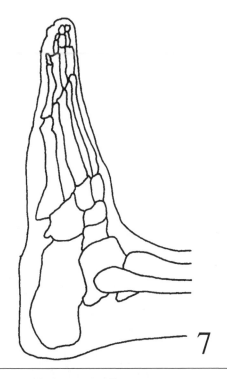

7

Anatomy and Physiology

Anatomy and Physiology

The goal of this chapter is twofold; (1) to present a physiological explanation of how reflexology works within the nervous system, and (2) to present an anatomical overview of how body parts work together reflexively.

How Does Reflexology Work?
Reflex Conditioning

"reflex;... Esp. Physiol. designating or of an involuntary action as a sneeze resulting when a stimulus is carried by an afferent (sensory) nerve to a nerve center and the response is reflected along an afferent (motor) nerve to some muscle or gland." Webster's Third World Dictionary, New York, Simon & Schuster, p. 1193.

It is a basic tenet of reflexology that the application of pressure to the feet has an effect on the whole body. Is there a physiological basis for such a belief? There is and it exists within the nervous system. A model for how reflexology works can be constructed from what we presently know about the nervous system. The physiological model presented here is based on the conditioning of reflexes.

The feet are sensory organs with a role in one of life's basic functions, locomotion. The ability to move about is crucial to survival, to gathering food and escaping from danger. Pressure sensors in the feet are a part of the body's reflexive network that makes possible a fight or flight response. In case of danger, the hands reach for a weapon, the feet prepare to fight or flee, and the internal organs provide adrenaline, oxygen, and glucose to fuel the effort. On a more mundane level, this same mechanism propels us through the day, taking us to work and moving us about our activities.

Locomotion is learned in infancy, but the learning never actually stops. We constantly receive feedback from the environment about where we are and what we are doing. The perception of pressure by the foot provides feed-back about what is underfoot. The demands of varying terrain call for the ability to ford a stream or stroll down a sidewalk. Such demands create a need for a response appropriate to the occasion.

Every day is not a new day for the foot or any other sensory organ. Using information gathered over a lifetime, instructions for sensory organs are preprogrammed in anticipation of events to come. The responses to our environment are preset programs of muscular tension fed forward to appropriate body parts from the brain. In other words, to continually respond to our changing environment, we need to receive feedback from our senses and to respond with "feed forward" directions from our brain. The classic example of a sensory organ receiving feed forward instructions occurs when a mother hears her infant cry. A mother can differentiate her own infant's crying from other infants because her hearing mechanism is tuned to her baby's cry. Thus specific instructions about that baby's cry are provided or fed forward by the brain.

It is this feed back / feed forward loop for sensory organs that makes possible a reflexology influence on the whole body. At the same time that a sensory organ such as the foot is being sent instructions from the brain, the internal organs are also receiving instructions. These instructions are about the levels of oxygen and fuel necessary to make movement possible. Although many parts of the brain are involved in this process, there is one final, common pathway in the brain stem that sends instructions to both the feet and the internal organs. The walking mechanism and the feet are, thus, inextricably linked to the internal organs.

The demands of walking call for an automatic, unconscious response to the ground underfoot. Changes in terrain call for changes within the reflexive response by the foot and the internal organs that fuel movement. For example, walking up a hill creates demands on the foot and the internal organs.

Any pressure perceived by the foot is a stimulus to which the entire body responds. Changes throughout the nervous system result from the perception of pressure by the foot. A discussion follows about the physiology of a pressure reflex and its role in the conditioning of the body.

Conditioning the Nervous System

"A conversation at a cocktail party will change your life," said Sir Charles Sherrington, neurologist and Nobel prize winner. It was not the content of the conversation to which he referred. It was the physical impingement of a voice on a nervous system that he considered. Sherrington was actually noting that, by definition, any sensory input changes the nervous system that perceives it.

A sensation of pressure from the foot travels from the skin inward along the route of the nervous system causing the body to adjust in a number of ways. Over time, continued exposure to pressure will cause these adjustments to be a more permanent fixture of the nervous system. The learning and conditioning that take place create a change in homeostasis or what the Russians referred to as brain-organ dynamics. The body, thus, alters its behavior and learns to act in the best manner possible.

From the Selye model, stress is a part of life. With only so much energy available to respond to stress, the best possible adaptation to stress is one that results in the least wear and tear on the body. New sensory input provides a break in the continuity of the established stress pattern. An interruption of the stress lessens its impact. Sensory input from the feet is of particular value because of the key role of the foot in survival.

Conditioning Change in the Nervous System

Conditioning change in the nervous system is possible because the foot plays an integral role in the survival function of locomotion. Patterns to cope with the stress of locomotion are formed in the foot itself, between body parts, and throughout the body as a whole. Those patterns of stress are:

Foot Stress: An overall tension level in the foot is necessary to maintain a readiness to walk and stand.

Reflex Stress: An overall tension level between body parts is necessary to integrate movement and the fuel needed to move.

Body Stress: A background level of tension is necessary to provide a continuous response to the internal and external environments.

The foot requires energy to make its contribution to locomotion. Too much energy expended in locomotion results in wear and tear throughout the body. The application of pressure techniques to the feet interrupts stress and creates the following changes in the nervous system:

Tension: Change in the overall body tone or stress level to create relaxation.

Body Image: Alteration of the body's picture of itself to create a more accurate perception.

Metabolic Rate: Changes in metabolism to create a more efficient response to stress.

Homeostasis, Brain / Organ Dynamics, Autonomic Regulation: By any name, changes in the overall operating balance of the body.

Circulation: Lymphatic and blood circulation is improved through physical application of technique.

The entire body adjusts in response to demands such as the stress of a pressure sensation. Each pressure sensory input alters the reflex image, the body image that is shared by all body parts. Adjustment is provided in the dynamic state of tension maintained to produce the best possible condition for the body and its functions. Reflexology utilizes pressure applied to a significant part of the body to interrupt stress and to create a break in routine that helps resolve the wear-and-tear aspect of stress.

Physiology of a Pressure Reflex

The following is a discussion of the stimulus of pressure and the response of the nervous system. Just as a road map leads one to a destination, pressure and the response to it travel along a well-established roadway in the nervous system.

N.B. Specific things happen when pressure is applied to the feet:
I. Stimulus: Information is sent from the foot to the brain.
II. Evaluation: The brain analyzes the information.
III. Response: The brain responds to the recent information by sending instructions to the entire body about how to adapt.

I. Stimulus

Proprioception: "Proprioceptive sensations are those that appraise the brain of the physical state of the body, including such sensations as 1. tension of the muscles, 2. tension of the tendons, 3. angulation of the joints, 4. deep pressure to the bottom of the feet." Arthur C. Guyton, Function of the Human Body, Philadelphia, W. B. Saunders, 1969, p. 272.

Proprioceptive Sensations

Proprioceptive sensations provide us with information about our body image; the stretch of muscle, the angulation of joints and deep pressure to the bottoms of the feet. Proprioception means literally, "to see oneself." Fine sensory gauges comprise the proprioceptive mechanism: (1) The Pacian corpuscles, such as those in the feet, sense deep pressure. They are the largest sensory receptors in the body, ranging in size from one to four millimeters. (2) Muscle stretch receptors in muscles and tendons sense stretch the amount

165

of stretch in the muscles and tendons. They thus provide information about muscle and joint movements and position.

Information from Pacian corpuscles (1) is linked to that of muscle stretch receptors. Because our body image and position are so critical to survival, such information travels to the brain on a fast-speed highway of information, the Epicritical nerve pathway.

Epicritical Nerve Pathway

The pressure nerve impulse is routed along the epicritical nerve pathway (2), thus pooling its information with other like (proprioceptive) information to begin the organization of the body imaging process. The epicritical nerve pathway gathers precise information critical to survival, such as touch, pressure, and position sense. The felt or perceived body image is constructed from this sensory information. The pat on the back can thus be quickly interpreted as being different from a poke in the eye.

Spinal Cord

The nerve impulse travels along the peripheral nervous system to the spinal cord (3). An exact representation of the body is organized in the spinal cord. Pieces of the picture are assembled from various body parts and projected in and up this pathway in an organized manner. Any basic reflex, such as the knee-jerk response, takes place on this level of the nervous system. After any reflexive response takes place, the information continues up the spinal cord to the brain. What the brain ultimately receives is a current picture of what is going on with respect to the surface of the body and where its body parts are. The brain organizes the responses (reflexive actions) that require a more sophisticated response than those of the spinal cord.

II. Evaluation

The Brain

At the brain stem (the medulla) (4), the nerve impulse crosses to the other half of the body. Sensory information about the left side of the body is thus reported to the right side of the brain. At this point the sensory information conveyed by the nerve impulse has entered the first of five different areas of the brain, all of which need information about pressure to perform a particular function.

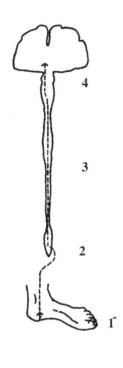

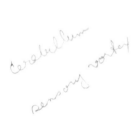

cerebellum
sensory cortex

Reflex Image in the Brain

The five areas of the brain serve as filters, each gleaning information necessary to further create a body image. Each is a specialist with a particular job, such as balance or fuel consumption, to consider. Each of the five has a template, a repeated body image. This is necessary for the complex task of receiving, processing, and responding to sensory information such as pressure in an orderly and appropriate manner. Comparing and contrasting new information with information on file takes place instantaneously. The repeated body images in the five areas of the brain serve as veritable filing cabinets. They store past experiences for comparison with present challenges.

The Brain Stem

The brain stem (4) provides a review of pressure information for any response requiring basic metabolic function such as respiration and circulation. Immediate response is necessary to alter breathing and blood flow.

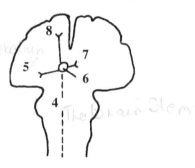

The brain stem is the body's switchboard for reflexively adjusting critical body functions. It is also referred to as the alarm clock of the brain. When you wake up in the morning, the brain stem answers two basic questions to show that a change has taken place between the sleeping state and the waking state: "Where am I?" and "What's to eat?" The first question has to do with the activity of getting up, and the second has to do with having the right amount of fuel to get to the breakfast table. The brain stem is signaling that a change has taken place. It acts as a coordinator of both incoming and outgoing messages, giving priority to the life support systems. Any information leaving the brain is routed through the brain stem, which serves as a volume control to adjust the body's tension level. It is the final common pathway for both the autonomic nervous system that regulates the internal organs and the motor nervous system that regulates muscle tone and movement.

Cerebellum

The cerebellum (5) is the balancer of body positions and movement. Without the cerebellum it would not be possible to make finely coordinated movements, such as balancing on a tightrope. It coordinates its efforts with the inner ear to keep us on our feet. A detailed pattern of sensory nerve information is routed to a specific site in the cerebellum. From the type of sensory information, such as pressure, and the body location, such as the foot, the cerebellum functions to create voluntary movement, finely-tuned movement, muscle tone, and balance. Thus, a soldier at attention maintains this posture because the cerebellum constantly provides the finely-tuned adjustments necessary to do so.

167

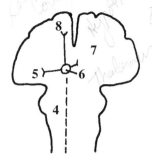

Thalamus

The thalamus (**6**) is the gatekeeper between the silent, unconscious parts of our brain and the consciously perceived parts of our brain. It links the lower centers of response (reflexes) and the higher levels of response (willed movement). The thalamus serves as a relay station to route the nerve impulse to conscious sensation (the cortex) and unconscious analysis (the hypothalamus). The nerve impulse is routed to a specific location of the thalamus that receives information about sensory type and body location, such as pressure and the foot.

The thalamus provides quick response to pain and then relays the information to the cortex to provide conscious perception of the pain. It is a relay system that works two ways. It takes unconscious information and turns it into conscious information. Then it takes conscious, willed information and turns it into unconscious reflexive action.

Hypothalamus

The hypothalamus (**7**) is a link between the nervous system and the endocrine glands. In response to the demand made by the nerve impulse, routed from the thalamus, the hypothalamus reflexively adjusts various metabolic rates. Hunger, thirst, fight, flight, and sex are all regulated by the hypothalamus, which also makes possible the physical activity needed to fulfill these basic motivational demands.

Cortex (Sensory)

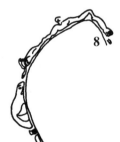

The nerve impulse is linked to conscious perception of sensation (of pressure, for example) in a particular part of the body (toe, for example) in a particular part of the sensory cortex (**8**). The cortex contains a mirror image of each and every body part that is referred to as the homunculous or "little man." Rather than being an exact representation of the body, the homunculous is a sensory map of the body. Each body part is represented according to how much sensory information it gathers. The lips and face, for example, cover a broad area of the sensory cortex whereas the trunk of the body occupies only a small section. The sensory cortex allows for point to point sensory perception and location. Pressure to the foot thus reports to a specific part of the sensory cortex.

The cortex is the most complex part of the nervous system and the highest integrating center. It separates the intelligence of humankind from that of an animal. Impulses at this level are thought to integrate the higher mental processes of thinking and memory. Perception, skilled behavior, and consciousness are all a part of cortex function. Focusing and learning new tasks take place in the cortex. For example, the goal of learning to shoot a basketball requires direction from the cortex.

III. Response

Cortex (Motor)

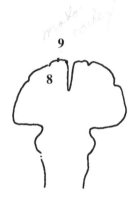

The sensation is now reflected from the sensory cortex to the motor cortex (9). The motor cortex has its own homunculous or orderly representation of body parts. Each muscle in the body has a representative area in the motor cortex that directs the activities of that muscle. Like the sensory cortex, the motor cortex is not proportional to the size of the body part but to the number of muscles and the skill executed by that body part. The hands and face have a larger representation than the trunk and legs.

If a muscle needs to be moved, the command comes from the motor cortex. Additional information is gathered from the cerebellum, the thalamus, and the hypothalamus to create a response to the nerve impulse. Response is projected through the reticular core in the brain stem to influence gland, organ, or muscle activity.

Autonomic Nervous System and Central Nervous System

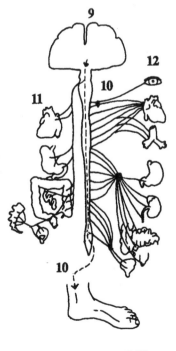

In case of danger, the brain communicates with the internal organs through the autonomic nervous system and the muscles, such as those of the foot, through the central nervous system. The reflexive response to a pressure stimulus also requires a response by the autonomic nervous system and the central nervous system.

The orderly flow of sensory information that flows to the brain after being evaluated flows back to every part of the body that requires this information. Now the brain "feeds forward" two sets of instructions. One set of instructions is for the readiness of the internal organs. The other set of instructions is for the level of muscular tension. (10) For these purposes detailed instructions project an image of the body back down the spinal cord and through cranial nerves to the entire nervous system. Instructions to the autonomic portion of the nervous system are relayed to the parasympathetic portion (11) by way of the cranial nerves emanating from the brain stem and instructions to the sympathetic portion (12) of the autonomic nervous system are projected through the reticular core, down the spinal cord to thoracic and lumbar they activate.

169

Instructions to the locomotor apparatus, such as the foot, (1) change existing background tone in pressure, stretch, and movement (proprioceptive) sensors and (2) create movement. Thus, the reflexive action created in response to a pressure sensation includes new instructions to the pressure sensor where the reflexive activity originated. Not only will the pressure sensor be changed by pressure but the whole body will also feel the influence.

Anatomy

It is a basic premise of reflexology that reflex areas on the feet are related to parts of the body. All are linked by the common goal of survival. Because of the need to react as a whole and to adapt to stress, an organized, team approach is utilized by the brain, internal organs, and all body parts to achieve the goal of survival. Wear-and-tear patterns emerge as a result of the demands of adapting to stress. These patterns tend to center on the systems of the body because of the organized response to stress, such as the "fight or flight response." These organs communicate with each other to accomplish a particular goal, such as breathing or digesting food. When a demand is placed on any of the systems, it tends to be reflected throughout the system.

Stress creates a pattern of response within the body. The following discussion of anatomy centers around the systems of the body. While each body part is listed separately, the goal is to present an image of all body parts working together for the whole.

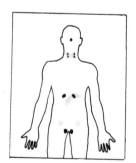

Endocrine System

Pituitary

Adrenal glands

Thyroid

Parathyroid

Pancreas

Reproductive

The endocrine glands serve as regulators. Together with the central nervous system they are responsible for controlling the complex activities of the body. Their messengers, the hormones, transmit their messages all over the body. There are many hormones serving many functions.

The endocrine glands are ductless, secreting their hormones directly into the bloodstream. These glands can malfunction either by being overactive (hyperactive) or underactive (hypoactive). Serious malfunction can result in such disorders as tetany, Addison's disease, diabetes, and dwarfism. Less critical malfunctions may result in subtle changes in the metabolism, physical and sexual development, mental well-being, and overall body health. As the reflexologist relieves stress (the source of many of these problems), the body is allowed to seek its own hormonal equilibrium.

Pituitary

Think of the endocrine glands as a large management team. The chief executive would be the pituitary. The pituitary gland is located at the base of the brain and is approximately one-half inch in diameter. It produces a number of hormones performing many different functions.

Functions

Affects hard and soft tissue growth. "Growth" can be defined as structural growth (such as body height). An imbalance in the pituitary can produce giantism or dwarfism. "Growth" can also be of soft tissue (such as tumors). The pituitary is involved in any type of growth, normal or abnormal.

growth

Metabolism is the rate at which cells work. The pituitary is the chief regulator, supervising the other glands involved in this process.

metabolism

The pituitary regulates the other endocrine glands, the arteries of the heart and body, water balance, blood pressure, sexual maturation, and reproduction.

regulation

Dysfunctions

Fever is a type of defensive reaction to protect the body. If the fever temperature of the body gets too high, its well-being is jeopardized. Together with the hypothalamus, the pituitary is involved in the body's attempt to cope with fever.

fever

The pituitary secretes a hormone called vasopressin, which regulates arterial constriction. Since fainting results from a sudden insufficient blood supply to the brain, this hormone and, thus, the pituitary are involved.

fainting

171

Thyroid Gland

The thyroid gland regulates the basal metabolism of the body cells. It is located in the front of the neck and is "H-shaped."

Functions

metabolism

Metabolism refers to the rate at which the body uses absorbed foods. It burns them to get heat and energy for its activities. Edema, overactivity, or underactivity cause obvious physical changes in weight as well as in physical and mental acuity. The thyroid produces thyroxine, a hormone which increases the rates of activity of almost all the chemical reactions in all the cells of the body.

growth and development

The thyroid produces a hormone that affects bone growth. It also controls calcium levels with calcitonin, a hormone that facilitates the movement of calcium into the bone. This operates in opposition to the parathyroid hormone, which increases the movement of calcium from the bone into the blood. The effect of the growth hormone of the pituitary gland is insignificant without the presence of thyroxine.

Dysfunctions

dryness of skin

The thyroid asserts control over skin health. An underactive thyroid can result in dryness of skin. The outer layer of the skin is a covering of dry, dead cells that are constantly being shed and replaced by cells from the growing layer. If the rate at which the cells being disposed of is abnormal, dryness of skin results. A deficiency of thyroid function directly controls this rate.

regulation

The thyroid does have an effect on the cholesterol level in the body. Cholesterol is a fatlike substance found in most tissues and is a main component of the lining of the arteries. If the level of cholesterol is too high, it can contribute to arteriosclerosis, or hardening of the arteries.

Parathyroid Glands

The parathyroids are embedded in the thyroid. Their hormone controls the levels of calcium and phosphorous in the blood. The level of calcium in the blood is important because it is involved in blood clotting, contraction of muscles, and the actions of the nerves. Most of the phosphorus in the body is combined with calcium in the bone, and the balance of assimilation and excretion of phosphorous is closely linked to that of calcium.

Functions

Bone is constantly being broken down and renewed. The parathyroid's job is to take calcium from this "reservoir" and add it to the body fluids when needed. The parathyroid can do its job properly only if the concentration of calcium in the body fluids is kept within very narrow limits.

calcium levels

Dysfunctions

Calcium and phosphorous are essential to the normal operation of the muscles and nerves. Parathyroid failure often causes an imbalance in calcium and phosphorous levels, which can result in muscle contractions, the serious form of which is called tetany.

cramps

Adrenal Glands

The adrenal glands are located on top of the kidneys. They have some fifty functions that interrelate with the other glands and are regulated by the pituitary.

Functions

Adrenaline is the "fight or flight" hormone. It stimulates heart action, releases glucose, raises the blood pressure, and increases the circulation of the blood to the muscles. It relaxes air passages, stimulates breathing, and prepares the body for action. In order to do this, it must slow down digestive and excretory processes, reducing the blood flow to all areas except the muscles and heart.

adrenaline production

The arterial, heart, and digestive muscles are involuntary in nature. The adrenal glands secrete hormones that have an effect on these muscles. For instance, peristalsis (wavelike contractions in the intestines) is necessary to propel the food along the digestive tract. The adrenal glands must maintain the muscle tone in the digestive tract to promote normal, healthy peristalsis.

muscle operation

The adrenal glands secrete hormones that control the water and mineral balances which, in turn affect the operations of the muscles.

water and mineral balance

Dysfunctions

Inflammation is a natural result of the body's attempt to heal itself. The adrenal glands produce a natural form of cortisone that aids in reducing inflammation. An injection of synthetic cortisone signals the adrenal glands

inflammation   that enough cortisone is in the system. Prolonged use of synthetic cortisone can thus inhibit the natural function of the glands themselves. Cortisone has other side effects as well.

stress   The adrenal glands help the body to combat stress. Cortisone prevents stress from becoming toxic to living tissue. Cortical hormones and adrenaline are main elements in the body's fight against fatigue. Fatigue lowers the body's ability to handle stress. (Stress is defined as injury, infection, environmental factors, psychological strain, etc.)

asthma   Because of the ability of adrenaline to open air passages, it is often administered in the treatment of asthma.

arthritis   Cortisone (see "Inflammation") is commonly used by the body to fight the inflammation associated with arthritis.

allergy   An allergic reaction is the body's response to the presence of certain types of food, clothing, or other physical matter in the immediate environment. Adrenaline and cortisone are two of the body's natural weapons against allergies.

low blood pressure   Blood pressure is the force exerted by the heart in pumping blood from its chambers. It is affected by the amount of adrenaline and noradrenaline produced by the adrenal glands. Adrenaline permits emergency contraction of some parts of the body and emergency relaxation of others. Noradrenaline is involved with contraction primarily and thus handles such jobs as the maintenance of proper blood pressure. Thus noradrenaline has an effect on long-term stress.

Pancreas

The pancreas lies mainly behind the stomach across the back of the abdomen. It is a dual-purpose organ with endocrine function (ductless: hormones are secreted directly into the bloodstream) and exocrine function (duct: digestive juices are secreted through the pancreatic duct).

Functions

digestion (exocrine)   Pancreatic juice is alkaline and neutralizes acid from the stomach. It has many enzymes which are catalysts that break down complex substances into simpler substances for absorption.

Insulin, a hormone produced by the pancreas, is essential in controlling the glucose level in the blood. Glucose is the principal energy food used by the body.

blood sugar level (endocrine)

Dysfunctions

Diabetes is a condition in which the pancreas fails to supply enough insulin to control the blood sugar (glucose) levels. There are many serious side effects and, unless sufficient insulin is supplied, diabetes can be fatal. The eyes and kidneys are usually the first to be affected if diabetes is not treated. This condition can occur during childhood as well as later in life. Juvenile diabetes is the more difficult and the more serious. Injections of insulin (or oral administration) and strict control of diet are common forms of treatment.

diabetes

Hypoglycemia is a condition in which the pancreas produces too much insulin, thereby creating a low blood sugar level. Many symptoms accompany a low blood sugar condition. For example, the brain has no fuel reserve except the supply of glucose in the blood. Hypoglycemia will impair the efficiency of the brain. It is principally through the regulation of diet that hypoglycemia is treated.

hypoglycemia

Reproductive Glands

All body cells require hormones just as all cells require nutrients. Virtually every cell in the body is affected by the hormones produced by the reproductive organs. The importance of the role these hormones play is felt throughout the human life cycle.

Functions

Sex hormones influence the reproductive capacities, maintain the sexual urge, and influence mental vigor and physical development.

sex hormones

Dysfunctions

The reproductive organs produce hormones used by the adrenal glands, and vice versa. This relationship may account for the effect the reproductive organs have in helping the body cope with allergies.

allergies

infertility   Dysfunction of the reproductive organs (i.e., low sperm count, blocked fallopian tube, irregular ovulation, suppressed sexual urge, etc.) results in the inability to conceive a child.

Digestive System

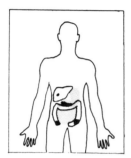

Liver

Gallbladder

Small Intestine

Ileocecal Valve

Large Intestine

The digestive system takes the complex molecules of food and breaks them down into simpler forms that are essential for the body's operations. The process starts with ingestion and ends with the disposal of the waste from the system. The digestive system is actually a long tube with various secretions from different organs being added along the way. The major organs considered here are the stomach, liver, gallbladder, pancreas, large and small intestines.

Stomach

The stomach is that part of the digestive tract located between the esophagus (food pipe) and the duodenum, the first portion of the small intestine. It is dilated and saclike in shape. The stomach is a neutral organ. Most of its common problems originate elsewhere.

Functions

digestion   During its two or three hour stay in the stomach, food is processed into a thin mash. With the exception of substances such as water and alcohol, no absorption of food takes place here. When food enters the stomach, the hormone gastrin is released into the blood to stimulate the secretion of gastric acids.

Dysfunctions

ulcer   A stomach ulcer is an open sore on the mucus membrane lining of the stomach. Emotional stress can promote the secretion of acid and is almost certainly a cause of stomach ulcers. Also, certain types of physical stress (e.g., extensive burns) can have the same effect.

176

Liver

The liver is the body's largest gland. It occupies the upper right and part of the upper left side of the abdominal cavity. It is essential to life.

Functions

During digestion the liver retains glycogen, a storable form of glucose, which enables it to supply a steady concentration to the blood, replacing what has been consumed as fuel. The brain keeps no stores at all and quickly dies if the supplies from the liver are cut off. The liver also stores proteins, fats, minerals, and vitamins for later use.

digestion

Bile is a secretion of the liver that helps break down the proteins, carbohydrates, and particularly the fats to prepare them for absorption into the blood system. Bile also lubricates the digestive tract.

bile

Dysfunctions

Poisoning of the liver is common because anything absorbed from the stomach is carried first to the liver for detoxification. The liver, therefore, gets a higher concentration of poisons than other organs. Many drugs and industrial chemicals can damage the liver during its attempt to protect the rest of the body. Alcohol is the most common of the poisons which the liver seeks to neutralize.

detoxification

Gallbladder

The gallbladder is embedded in the liver. It acts as a storehouse for the bile, releasing it as needed.

Functions

Bile accumulates in the gallbladder until after a heavy meal. Fats stimulate the secretion of the bile. Its active functions depend on bile salts formed in the liver from cholesterol. This emulsifies the fat, making it easy to digest.

bile storage

Dysfunctions

Fat particles, particularly cholesterol, can crystallize from the bile, forming gallstones in the gallbladder.

gallstones

Small Intestines

The beginning of the small intestine is the "C-shaped" duodenum, where the digestion of food is brought near completion. The remainder of the small intestine is a long, narrow tube (22.5 ft.) lined with a vast number of small, fingerlike projections called villi, which absorb the nutrients from the digested food.

Functions

peristalsis

Peristalsis is the wavelike contraction of the muscles of the intestines, which propels the food along the digestive tract.

absorption

Nutrients are absorbed by the villi of the small intestines and then "pumped" out to the blood and lymph vessels leading from the villi.

Ileocecal Valve

The ileocecal valve is a passageway between the small and large intestine. Its principal function is to prevent backfill of the contents from the colon into the small intestine.

Dysfunctions

mucus control

Mucus is a clear fluid forming a protective barrier on the surfaces of the lining of membranes. The area around the ileocecal valve is responsible for the control of mucus. If the mucus is not controlled properly, it can break up and be absorbed into the digestive system. Mucus control is important in related conditions such as sinus problems and lung problems.

Large Intestines

The large intestine is much wider than the small intestine and is about five feet long. It consists of the ascending, transverse, and descending colon (including sigmoid and rectum).

Functions

absorption

The colon absorbs water and electrolytes from the waste material.

storage

The colon stores fecal matter until it can be expelled.

Urinary System

Kidneys

Ureter Tubes

The urinary system is comprised of the kidneys, ureter tubes, and the bladder. It is the chief disposal unit of the body.

Kidneys

The kidneys are the chief organs of the urinary system, located about the midback. They perform many functions related to regulating fluid in the body and purifying the blood.

Functions

Filtration in the kidneys begins with the straining of fluid from the blood. This fluid is then separated into waste products to be excreted and vital substances to be reabsorbed.

chief eliminator

The kidneys regulate the acid/alkaline balance of the body's other fluids; they stimulate the production of red blood cells when needed; they watch over the amounts of salts and other substances in the blood.

Ureter Tubes

The ureter tubes are the link between the kidneys and the bladder. They are narrow elastic passageways through which urine passes after being produced in the kidneys.

Bladder

The bladder acts as a reservoir. When it is full of urine, nerve fibers react to initiate urination.

The Circulatory System

In a general sense, the circulatory system is responsible for the constant flow of blood and other body fluids. The heart is a pump whose action keeps the blood circulating, carrying nutrients, hormones, vitamins, antibodies, heat, and oxygen to the tissues and taking away all waste materials. The circulatory system consists of the heart, blood vessels (arteries, veins, capillaries), and the lymphatic system. The lymphatic system acts as an auxiliary to the venous system.

The Heart

The heart is the most amazing pump in the world. Every day it beats about one hundred thousand times, pumping the equivalent of eighteen hundred gallons of blood through some sixty thousand miles of blood vessels. It is a hollow, muscular organ in the chest – no bigger than a clenched fist.

Functions

The sole function of the heart is to pump blood from the veins into the arteries.

Lungs

Each lung is a network of hollow tubes and sacs that remove oxygen from the air in exchange for carbon dioxide. The lungs are located above the diaphragm in the chest. Breathing is effected when the diaphragm muscle pulls down, enlarging the chest cavity and causing air to be drawn into the lungs.

The Lymphatic System

Spleen

Thymus

Lymphatic Nodes

Lymphatic Drain

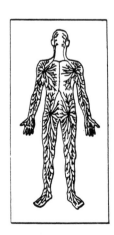

The lymphatic system is a network of thin-walled vessels found in all parts of the body except the central nervous system. These vessels contain the lymph fluid, which bathes all of the body's cells, feeding them with the nutrients removed by the small intestine. The fluid is filtered through little balls of cells called lymph nodes. These nodes are located mainly in the groin, armpit, and neck.

Functions

The lymph nodes are small "fortresses" where the lymph fluid deposits bacteria or foreign matter for disposal. In the nodes the infectious material is encapsulated and ingested by lymphocytes, which produce antibodies. These antibodies are the body's chief defense against infection.

fighting infection

The lymphatic system works in partnership with the venous system to effectively transport wastes produced by cell metabolism. Large particles, such as old debris of dead tissues, protein molecules, and dead bacteria, cannot pass from the tissues directly into the blood through the small pores of the capillaries. The lymphatic is an accessory system taking care of those materials.

waste removal

Dysfunctions

The lymph fluid is not pumped throughout the body by any heartlike organ but is pressed forward by contractions of surrounding muscles. Lymph fluid can pool in the legs and feet, which then swell. This pooling can be caused by a plugged lymph node, heart disorder, too much salt in the diet, or as a side effect of medication.

edema

Spleen

The spleen, an organ in the abdomen cupping the left edge of the pancreas, is part of the lymphatic system.

Functions

The spleen produces antibodies and filters the lymph fluids in lymphocytes the same way as a lymph node.

manufacturing lymphocytes

The spleen removes and destroys faulty or deformed red blood cells and recycles iron for hemoglobin production. Hemoglobin is the substance that carries oxygen to the tissues. The spleen also is a reservoir for the storage of extra blood.

blood cell quality control

Dysfunctions

The spleen is involved in various widespread disorders of the lymphoid and blood-forming tissues; e.g., leukemia, Hodgkin's disease, and anemia.

Thymus

The thymus is a lymph gland located behind the upper part of the breastbone.

Functions

maturation and development of the immune system

The thymus plays a key role in the development of the immune system in infants. It appears to continue to play an important part in the body's immune system throughout life.

The Lymphatic Drain

The lymphatic system drains its fluid into two veins at the base of the neck. These veins are important for the transition of the lymph fluid into the venous system. The waste and excess fluid is removed from the blood by the kidneys and eliminated by urination.

The Central Nervous System

The nervous system, in general, regulates rapid muscular and secretory activities of the body, whereas the hormonal system (endocrine) regulates mainly the slowly reacting metabolic functions. The central nervous system consists of the brain, spinal cord, and the nerves emanating from them.

The Brain and the Cranial Nerves

The brain consists of two hemispheres. The left controls the right half of the body and vice versa. This "crossover" is important to the reflexologist in that it is the major exception to zone theory. In zone theory the right foot represents the right half of the body, and the left foot, the left half. Disorders involving one side of the brain will appear as a dysfunction on the opposite side of the body. In the case of a stroke, for example, the large toe on the opposite side from the paralysis will be more sensitive.

The brain is the central computer that controls both the voluntary and the involuntary systems of the body. In other words it controls the central nervous system and the endocrine system, both of which jointly control the complex activities of the whole body.

There are twelve pairs of cranial nerves arising from the brain and passing through the holes in the skull. Some of the cranial nerves are only sensory (taste, smell, sight, and hearing), but the majority are motor nerves. Probably the most important of the cranial nerves is the vagus nerve. It is the largest nerve in the body, supplying the heart, lungs, and abdominal organs.

Spinal Cord and Spinal Nerves

The spinal cord is the continuation of the brain below the skull. It is a column of nerve tissue enclosed in the spinal canal, a tunnel in the backbone. The nerves originating from the spinal cord are channels for conveying information from the peripheral nerves of the body to the muscles and glands.

The cervical nerves control the neck and arms. The thoracic portion provides nerves to the chest. The lumbar nerves are distributed to the lower extremities, the legs and feet, and the sacral nerves mainly supply the organs of the pelvis, and the pelvic and buttock muscles.

The spinal nerves are named and numbered according to the vertebral divisions of the spinal column into cervical, thoracic, lumbar, and sacral segments. Each division has an effect on a region of the body.

The spine has seven cervicals. From the seventh cervical down are the twelve thoracic vertebrae, each carrying a pair of ribs. These end at the waistline, which marks the beginning of the five lumbar vertebrae. This is the lower back. The lower back has a profound effect on everything in that region, such as the reproductive organs, digestive tract, and the lower limbs. Below the lumbar vertebrae are five fused vertebrae that form the sacrum and the vestiges of the tail, the coccyx. This area can affect many parts of the body, including the head (headaches).

The Head

The head accommodates the brain, several sense organs, and inlets for air and food.

The Ears

The ears gather the vibrations from the air and turn them into meaningful messages. The outer shell of the ear only captures the sound. The actual mechanism for hearing is well protected in the head. The sound travels down a tunnel into the middle ear, which is enclosed in a membrane called the eardrum. The eardrum flutters in response to sound. A fine set of bones called the hammer, anvil, and stirrup are attached to the inside of the eardrum. The eardrum vibrations make these bones move in response, transmitting their message to the inner ear. The inner ear houses apparatuses for two separate functions. The cochlea takes the vibrations and translates them into nerve messages. The semicircular canals housed within the cochlea are responsible for maintaining balance.

The Eyes

The eyes act like a camera, taking in the view and sending the message to the brain. A lens focuses light into the eye. The light travels to the back of the eye, shining on a fine nerve network of cells called the retina. The retina triggers a signal of what it sees to the optic nerve. The message is relayed through the second cranial nerve to the brain, where it is interpreted.

Muscular System

Muscle is the most abundant tissue in the body. It accounts for some two fifths of the body's weight. There are two involuntary types of muscles: the smooth muscles (found in the walls of the digestive and the urinary tract, other hollow organs, and the blood vessels) and the cardiac muscles (muscles of the heart). The striated muscles are voluntary muscles, but they also take part in unconscious reflexes. Muscles essentially have two actions: contraction and relaxation. The range of these two actions is important for the body's return to equilibrium. Chemicals essential in contracting the muscles to meet certain challenges can be left over, causing residual tension. Residual tension in these muscles can have effects on the skeletal system, organs, glands, and circulatory system.

Skeletal System

The bones of the body are not a static structure. They store nearly all of the body's reserves of calcium. They also manufacture red blood cells (a function performed by red bone marrow). The skeleton provides a firm framework, giving shape to the body and its parts. It supports and protects vital parts such as the heart, brain, and lungs from injury. The skeleton facilitates body movements by acting in cooperation with various muscles attached to the bones by tendons.

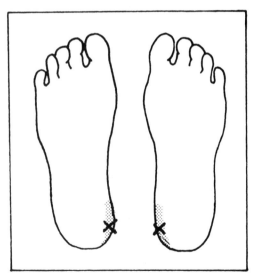

8

Directory of Protocols

Directory of Protocols

A key component of reflexology work is the selection of reflex areas to which technique is applied. Reflex areas are selected within general guidelines. In brief, the choice is one of reflex areas reflecting body parts that best impact the cause of the stress related disorder.

Reflex area influence

Reflexology technique application is directed at reflex area(s) that reflect the body part(s) central to the cause of the disorder. Appropriate technique application to, for example, the kidney reflex area is seen to effect the function and structure of the kidney.

Stress related influence

Stress is seen as a basic cause of many disorders. Technique is applied to the solar plexus reflex area to prompt relaxation. Application of dessert techniques serve to boost feelings of relaxation.

Function-related reflex area influence

Technique is applied to the reflex area(s) of the body part, organ or system whose function impacts the condition reported by the client. A report of asthma concerns, for example, is met with application of technique to not only the lung reflex areas but also the adrenal gland reflex areas to prompt a response by the adrenal glands.

Relationship within body systems influence

All organs within a body system influence each other. For example, a concern related to the kidney includes technique application to the reflex areas of all organs of the urinary system, the kidney reflex area as well as bladder and ureter reflex areas.

Zonal relationship influence

Technique is applied to all reflex areas within a zone. For example, an eye concern includes technique applied to the eye reflex area as well as reflex areas in the second zone such as the kidneys.

Referral area influence

In cases of injury foot or ankle injury, technique is applied to the referral area. Thus, technique is not applied to an injured ankle but is applied to the referral area for the ankle, the wrist. For other referral relationships, the reflexologist demonstrates self-help techniques to be applied by the client.

Targeted Session

The goal of the reflexologist is to efficiently and effectively apply technique to the foot. The question is, How can the reflexologist best elicit the relaxation response so that the individual feels a change in stress level? Ideally, technique is applied to the whole foot and, then, technique is applied to the foot a second time targeting areas of emphasis.

When a limited amount of time is available for a session (15 minutes or less), a shortened, targeted session consists of technique applied to each foot: a series of desserts, technique application to the reflex areas of emphasis, and a series of desserts. In addition, technique is always applied to the kidney reflex area. For example:

Arrhythmia (Example of targeted session)

Apply technique to the left foot.			
Reflex areas	**Side to side**	**Metatarsal mover**	**Brain stem**
Heart	**Adrenal gland**	**Kidney**	**Lung press**
Apply technique to the right foot.			

Index of Protocols

Indicates Controlled Study. See pp. 158-160.

Directory of Protocols

The Directory of Protocols shows the selection of reflex areas for technique applications to stress-related disorders. Protocols are listed by systems of the body to demonstrate both the commonalities of reflex area selection within a system and the differences in selections. Information includes (1) disorder, (2) reflex areas selected for technique emphasi, (3) illustration of selected reflex areas, and (4) a description of the disorder to provide information about the cause of the disorder.

Cardio-vascular System

The guidelines utilized in reflex area selection reflect the cause of the disorder, i. e. brain stem functioning in arrhythmia as opposed to solar plexus in hypertension. Selection includes: reflex area influences (heart, chest region, midback), and function-related reflex area. influences (adrenal glands, brain stem, solar plexus, liver, thyroid, pituitary).

Disorder	Reflex Areas	Quick Reference
Angina-Pectoris (See "Research")	Heart (p. 48) Adrenal glands (p. 53) Chest (p. 48) Lymphatic drain (pp. 49-51) Midback (p. 59) Kidney (p. 51, p. 54)	

Angina is a pain in the chest caused by a spasm of the coronary arteries of the heart. Work through the heart reflex area thoroughly on both the tops and bottoms of both feet. Pay particular attention to the troughs between the first and second toes. Target the tension level with the special emphasis of dessert technique technique application to the ball of the foot. Explore the big toe and its joints for touch stress cues.

Arrhythmia	Brain stem (p. 59) Heart (p. 48) Adrenal glands (p. 53) Kidneys (p. 49, p. 54)	

Arrhythmia is an abnormal heart rhythm. In an arrhythmia, the heartbeats may be too slow (tachycardia), too rapid (bradycardia), too irregular (atrial fibrillation and ventricular fibrillation), or too early. Technique application to the brain stem and adrenal gland reflex areas recognize the roles of those body parts in regulating heart beat.

189

Cholesterol levels (See "Research")	Liver (pp. 43-46) Pancreas (pp. 41-43) Kidneys (p. 51, p. 54) Brain stem (p. 58)	

Cholesterol is a critically important molecule essential to the formation of: bile acids (which aid in the digestion of fats), Vitamin D, Progesterone, Estrogens (estradiol, estrone, estriol), Androgens (androsterone, testosterone) Mineralocorticoid hormones (aldosterone, corticosterone), and Glucocorticoid hormones (cortisol). Cholesterol is also necessary for the normal permeability and function of cell membranes. Cholesterol is carried in the bloodstream as lipoproteins. Low-density lipoprotein (LDL) cholesterol is the "bad" cholesterol because elevated LDL levels are associated with an increased risk of coronary artery (heart) disease. Conversely, high-density lipoprotein (HDL) cholesterol is the "good" cholesterol since high HDL levels are associated with less coronary disease. Although some cholesterol is obtained from the diet, most cholesterol is made in the liver and other tissues. The pancreas impacts metabolism of fats. The kidneys are involved in blood circulation that increases as fatty deposits adhere to artery walls. Thus, all three organs are targeted with reflexology work to impact cholesterol levels.

Congestive heart failure	Heart / lung (p. 48) Kidneys (p. 51, p. 54) Adrenal glands (p. 53)	

With congestive heart failure, the heart loses its ability to pump blood effectively. As a result blood may back up in other areas of the body; the liver, the gastro-intestinal tract and extremities (right-sided failure) and the lungs (left-sided heart failure). Hypertension and coronary artery disease are the most frequent causes of congestive heart failure. Reflex areas targeted with reflexology work include heart/lung, liver, and the digestive system.

Heart Attack	Heart / lung (p. 48) Adrenal glands (p. 53) Sigmoid colon (p. 56) Kidneys (p. 49, p. 54)	

A heart attack occurs due to an obstruction of the coronary artery or one of its branches by a blood clot, depriving part of the heart muscle of blood. The heart reflex area extends across the ball of the left foot and onto part of the right foot as well. The entire ball of the foot needs emphasis. Note any touch stress cues on the top of the foot in the chest / lung reflex area, especially in the third zone. The heart is a muscle, and the adrenal gland reflex area can help with muscle tone. The sigmoid colon is one part of the intestine particularly prone to the trapping and pocketing of gas. This increased pressure can back up along the colon to the transverse section, where it can put pressure on the chest cavity. Note the touch stress cue of thickening or hardening around the bunion joint.

Hypertension / Atherosclerosis (See "Research")	Solar plexus (p. 47) Adrenal glands (p. 53) Kidneys (p. 51, p. 54) Pituitary (p. 41) Liver (pp. 43-46) Thyroid (p. 41)	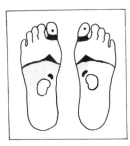

Hypertension is a condition in which the heart is forced to pump under higher pressure, which puts excessive strain on it. Hypertension can speed up the development of atherosclerosis (blockage of arteries). When arteries supplying the brain are blocked, a stroke can result. When the blocked arteries are those that supply the heart, a heart attack can result. Atherosclerosis is often referred to as "hardening of the arteries." Tension causes the blood pressure to rise, forcing materials such as cholesterol into the walls of the arteries. Naturally, as these materials build up, blood flow is further restricted, and the kidneys seek to compensate by releasing a hormone whose job is to increase the blood pressure. Then more materials are forced into the vessel walls and the cycle continues.

The solar plexus reflex area is worked for tension reduction. The adrenal glands are the key endocrine glands for meeting stress, both short and long term. Work liver and thyroid reflex areas to address cholesterol concerns. Brain stem and hypothalamus reflex areas are included for their regulatory roles.

Phlebitis	Liver (pp. 43-46) Adrenal glands (p. 53) Kidneys (p. 51, p. 54) Lymphatic / groin (p. 61) Knee / leg (p. 60)	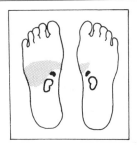 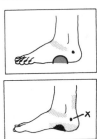

Phlebitis is an inflammation usually associated with blockage of a vein by a blood clot. The liver is involved in the clotting mechanism and is a helpful reflex area to work on the feet. The part of the arm corresponding to the affected part of the leg (referral area) is a valuable tool for reaching the problem through self-help technique application. Do not work on the affected area itself. Working the adrenal gland reflex area helps with the inflammation. If phlebitis is active, request the doctor's permission before proceeding with reflexology work.

Digestive System

The guidelines utilized in reflex area selection include: reflex area influences (colon, liver/gallbladder, stomach, tailbone, lower back) and function-related influences (adrenal glands, solar plexus, endocrine glands).

Colitis	Colon (pp. 53-57) Solar plexus (p. 43) Adrenal glands (p. 53)	

Colitis is an inflammation of the colon. It is important to find on the foot the area that relates to the irritation in the colon. Take note of the touch stress cue of thickening in the reflex area. Tension is often involved in digestive problems. Work the solar plexus reflex area for tension and the adrenal gland reflex area for inflammation. Note any protrusion of the bone on the outside of the foot (base of the fifth metatarsal). Take particular note of this visual stress cue if it is red and inflamed.

Constipation (See "Research")	Colon (pp. 53-57) Liver / gallbladder (pp. 43-46) Adrenal glands (p. 53) Solar plexus (p. 43) Lower back (p. 56, p. 60)	

Constipation arises from a variety of sources, including tension. The liver and gallbladder produce and store the bile needed for digestion. The adrenal glands are essential to smooth muscle operation, as in the peristaltic (muscle) contraction of the digestive system. Problems in the lower back can affect everything within its area. The digestive system is also vulnerable to the side effects of tension. The reflex areas on the feet corresponding to these parts of the body should be worked. Note any protrusion of the base of the fifth metatarsal. Take particular note of the visual stress cue if it is red and inflamed.

Diverticulitis	Colon (pp. 53-57) Sigmoid colon (p. 56) Solar plexus (p. 47) Adrenal glands (p. 53)	

The diverticulum is a sac arising from the bowel wall. Diverticulitis is the condition in which this sac becomes inflamed. This disorder is fairly common around the lower colon area. Work the entire colon reflex areas on the feet, paying particular attention to the sigmoid colon reflex area. Work the adrenal gland reflex area for inflammation. Note any protrusion of the bone on the outside of the foot (base of the fifth metatarsal). Take particular note of this stress cue if it is red and inflamed. Note the touch stress cue of thickening in the colon reflex area.

Dyspepsia (See "Research")	Stomach (pp. 43-46) Solar plexus (p. 47)	

Upper abdominal symptoms of dyspepsia may include pain or discomfort, bloating, feeling of fullness with very little intake of food (early satiety), a feeling of unusual fullness following meals (postprandial fullness), nausea, loss of appetite, heartburn, regurgitation of food or acid, and belching. The term dyspepsia is often used for these symptoms when they are not typical of a well-described disease, for example, gastrointestinal reflux (GERD), and the cause is not clear. Once a cause for the symptoms has been determined, the term dyspepsia usually is dropped for a more specific diagnosis, e.g., gastric ulcer, gastrointestinal reflux (GERD). The stomach and solar plexus reflex areas are targeted.

Flatulence	Sigmoid colon (p. 56) Solar plexus (p. 47) Colon and small intestine (pp. 53-57)	

Flatulence is an excessive accumulation of gas in the stomach or intestine. The sigmoid colon, because of its location, is a prime target for flatulence. On the feet, the sigmoid colon, the intestines, and the solar plexus reflex areas should be worked. Note any protrusion of the bone on the outside of the foot (base of the fifth metatarsal). Take particular note of this cue if it is red and inflamed. Work the heels thoroughly. Apply desserts that move and stretch the ankle (see pp. 36-38).

Gallstones	Liver / gallbladder (pp. 43-46)	

Gallstones are crystallized fatty particles, particularly cholesterol. The size of a gallstone can be as small as a seed to as large as a lemon. The larger the gallstone, the greater the potential for problems. Work the liver / gallbladder reflex areas thoroughly. Apply finger walking technique to the top of the foot. Note any sensitivity cue in zones four and five. Be aware of the potential for hypersensitivity.

Hemorrhoids	Tailbone (p. 60) Hip region (p. 60) Lower back (p. 56, p. 60) Sigmoid colon (p. 56) Solar plexus (p. 43)	

Hemorrhoids are varicose veins of the rectum. At times the colon itself actually becomes extended outward. Work the lower back / tailbone reflex area. This includes all the areas around the heel (particularly where the shoe meets the back of the foot). The bottom of the heels, particularly the sigmoid colon reflex area, can be of value. Tension may be part of the problem. Work the solar plexus reflex area. Observe the stress cues, and apply technique to the heels and lower back, hip/back/sciatic reflex areas, as well as the ankle. Note stress cue of protrusion on the side of the foot.

Hiatal Hernia	Solar plexus (p. 47) Adrenal glands (p. 53)	

A hernia of the diaphragm may occur at the opening through which the esophagus passes. It is a ballooning of the diaphragm wall. The diaphragm is a strong layer of muscle and fibrous tissue dividing the chest and the abdominal cavities. People often complain of indigestion because a spasm in the sphincter valve leading to the stomach allows acid to splash up into the unprotected esophagus. The esophagus runs to the left as it enters the stomach, so the left foot will tend to be more sensitive than the right in the solar plexus reflex area. Sharp pain will often be encountered here. Work the diaphragm/solar plexus reflex area completely, emphasizing the adrenal gland reflex area for muscle tone. Make a press and assess evaluation of the solar plexus reflex area.

Ulcer	Stomach (pp. 51-53) Solar plexus / Diaphragm (p. 43) Adrenal glands (p. 53) Colon (pp. 54-57) Endocrine glands	

An ulcer is a persistent break in the skin or mucus membrane that fails to heal. Circulation is not functioning in the area. There are many types and locations of ulcers, the most common of which is in the stomach. The solar plexus reflex area can help with stress-related disorders, although not all ulcers are associated with stress. Working the adrenal gland reflex area helps with stress as well as assisting with the inflammation. Work the stomach reflex area on the feet (gastric ulcer). Note the touch stress cue of thickening or hardening in the stomach reflex area.

Ear

The guidelines utilized in reflex area selection include influences: reflex area (eye / ear) and function-related (adrenal glands, shoulder, neck).

Earache	Eye / ear (pp. 46-47) Shoulder (pp. 48-49) Adrenal glands (p. 53)	

Infection is a prime cause of earache. Note the stress cue of sensitivity in the toes. Work the eye/ear reflex areas thoroughly, giving added emphasis to the adrenal gland reflex areas when inflammation or infection is involved. Note the touch stress cue of thickening in the eye/ear reflex area.

Hearing Disorders	Eye / ear (pp. 46-47) Neck (p. 58)	

Partial or complete loss of hearing may be due to age, accident, genetic defect, occupational hazard, or other cause. The bones of the middle ear are vital, and if damaged, little can be done to improve the hearing. Balance is still an important function of the ear, even when hearing is impaired or lost. As with any hearing problem, technique should be applied to the eye/ear and neck reflex areas. Note the touch stress cue of thickening or hardening in the ear reflex area.

Tinnitus	Eye / ear (pp. 46-47) Neck (p. 58) Adrenal glands (p. 53) Shoulder (pp. 48-50)	

Tinnitus is a ringing, buzzing, or hissing in the ear. It can arise from any disorder of the ear or of the auditory nerve. Wax in the ear, blockage of the Eustachian tube, and irritation of the auditory nerve are the most common causes.

Work the eye/ear and neck reflex areas completely. Technique is applied to the adrenal gland reflex area for possible infection in the Eustachian tube. Note the touch stress cue of thickening or hardening in the ear reflex area.

196

Endocrine System

The guidelines utilized in reflex area selection include: reflex area influences (pancreas, pituitary, thyroid, adrenal glands) and function-related influences (liver, spine).

Diabetes **Hypoglycemia** (See "Research")	Pancreas (pp. 51-53) Pituitary (p. 41) Thyroid (p. 42) Liver (pp. 51-53) Adrenal glands (p. 53)	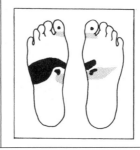 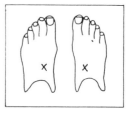

Diabetes is a disease characterized by the body's inability to burn up sugars (carbohydrates) that have been consumed. An insufficient production of insulin is responsible. Insulin is a hormone produced by cells in the pancreas, which secretes insulin into the blood, permitting the metabolism and utilization of sugar. If this secretion is insufficient, the blood sugar level rises rapidly, causing a series of dangerous conditions. The reverse of this condition is hypoglycemia. Frequent urination (an attempt to rid the blood of excess glucose), loss of weight (an attempt to burn fat instead of glucose), and degeneration of small vessels (particularly in the eyes and kidneys) are symptomatic of diabetes. It can lead to blindness and kidney disease. Circulatory problems frequently complicate this condition. Juvenile diabetes is the severe form of this disease.

Hypoglycemia is a deficiency of sugar in the blood. There are many interrelated systems that keep this level constant, despite large changes in the consumption or expulsion of glucose (blood sugar). All carbohydrates are converted to glucose. Glucose is stored in the form of glycogen in the liver and muscles. When glucose is needed, it is removed from the glycogen storehouses. A variety of exotic hormones maintain the balance between the combustion of glucose and its storage. Insulin is the most important hormone in this process. (See "Diabetes.") Hypoglycemia is characterized by too much insulin in the blood. It removes glucose from the blood by increasing combustion, and thus it increases the amount of glycogen in storage. This is at the expense of the blood.

There are many symptoms of hypoglycemia. Sudden drops in energy levels and mental depression are often signs of this disorder. It can impair the efficiency of the brain, which depends on a constant supply of blood sugar because it has no stores of its own. Careful working of the pancreas reflex areas on both the right and left foot is necessary. The adrenal glands are involved because of their regulation of the storage of proteins, carbohydrates, and fats. The liver is a storehouse and regulator for glycogen. The thyroid and pituitary play a role in metabolism and therefore are involved in this process. Working all the endocrine gland reflex areas is helpful.

Pancreatitis	Pancreas (pp. 51-53) Gall bladder (pp. 51-53) Liver (pp. 51-53) Adrenal glands (p. 53)	

Panreatitis is an inflammation of the pancreas. Of the many diverse causes of pancreatitis, the most common are alcoholism, disease of the gallbladder or via virus. The gall bladder could be the source. Adrenal glands are involved in inflammation. Technique is applied to the reflex areas of these organs.

Thyroid disorders	Thyroid (p. 42) Pituitary (p. 41) Adrenal glands (p. 53)	

Goiter, hypothyroidism or hyperthyroidism causing an inability of the thyroid to produce sufficient hormones thyrotrophic hormone and thyroxin resulting a lower metabolic rate (hypothyroidism) or increased metabolic rate (hyperthyroidism). In addition, the thyroid plays a role in heart and cholesterol disorders. Technique is applied to the reflex areas of these organs.

Eye

The guidelines utilized in reflex area selection include influences: reflex area (eye / ear) and function-related (neck) and zonal (kidneys). Eye reflex areas include the stems and bases of the toes.

Eye Disorders	Eye / ear (pp. 46-47) Neck (p. 58) Kidneys (p. 51, p. 54)	

Apply technique to the eye / ear reflex areas at the stems and bases of the toes. The neck reflex area is a good helper area to eye stress because the blood and nerve supply passes through it. Because of the zonal relationship, the kidney reflex areas provide additional aid. Note the touch stress cues of thickening, hardening, and sensitivity in the eye reflex areas.

Atrophy of the Optic Nerve	Eyes (pp. 46-47) Kidneys (p. 51, p. 54) Neck (p. 58)	

Atrophy of the optic nerve, a degeneration of the nerve fibers, occurs for a variety of reasons. A loss of vision results. Note the stress cues of thickening, hardening, and sensitivity in the balls of the toes and on the tops of the toes.

Cataracts	Eye / ear (pp. 46-47) Kidneys (p. 51, p. 54) Neck (p. 58)	

Cataracts are growths over the lens of the eye; the lens becomes opaque. Cataracts generally occur in old age, they but can also occur as a result of injury. In rare cases cataracts may be present at birth. The earlier they are detected, the better the chances for successful treatment. The eye/ear reflex areas need thorough attention. When the lens becomes totally grown over and surgery becomes necessary, it is still important to work the eye/ear area and other associated areas. This assists the healing process and helps control the scarring that accompanies surgery. Since these areas lie in the same zones as the kidney areas, use each as a referral area to help the other. Tension in the neck can also cause eye/ear problems. Work the neck areas thoroughly. Technique applied to the ball of the foot and the toes can be helpful. Check for stress cues, especially hard tonus, in the eye reflex areas.

Detached Retina	Eye / ear (pp. 46-47) Neck (p. 58) Kidneys (p. 51, p. 54)	

199

The separation of the retina from the outer layers of the eyeball will result in partial or total blindness. Explore the joint of the big toe for touch stress cues. Evaluate the big toe with a press and assess observation.

Glaucoma	Eye / ear (pp. 46-47) Neck (p. 58) Kidneys (p. 51, p. 54)	

Glaucoma is an eye disease associated with increased pressure of the fluid in the eyeball, leading to blindness if left untreated. Note the touch stress cue of thickening or hardening in the eye/ear reflex area. As with all eye stress, technique application to the neck and kidney reflex areas on the feet should be emphasized.

Macular degeneration	Eye (pp. 46-47)	

A disease that affects the macula, the part of the eye responsible for central vision, and impairs central vision. The macula is in the center of the retina at the back of the eye. As we read, light is focused onto the macula where millions of cells change the light into nerve signals that travel to the brain and tell it what we are seeing. This is our central vision. With normal central vision, we are able to read, drive, and perform other activities that require fine, sharp, straight-ahead vision. Macular degeneration rarely causes blindness because only the center of vision is affected. However, injury to the macula in the center of the retina can destroy the ability to see straight ahead clearly and sometimes make it difficult to read, drive, or perform other daily activities that require fine central vision. Work is applied to the eye reflex areas as well as the second joints of the second and third toes.

Immune System

The guidelines utilized in reflex area selection include: reflex area influences (lymphatic glands) and function-related influences (adrenal glands, reproductive organs, pituitary).

AIDS	Lymphatic system (p. 61) Endocrine glands Brain (pp. 43-46) Pancreas (pp. 51-53) Liver (pp. 51-53)	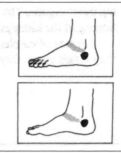 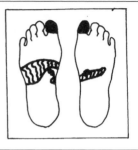

Acquired immunodeficiency disease (AIDS) is a disease caused by infection with the human immunodeficiency virus (HIV). Technique is applied to the lymphatic glands reflex areas are important to combat the virus, endocrine glands reflex areas to boost the immune response and the pancreas reflex area to combat pancreatitis, a common side effect to AIDS.

Allergies	Adrenal glands (p. 53) Reproductive glands (pp. 62-63) Pituitary (p. 41)	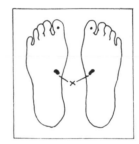 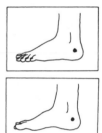

An allergic response is a misuse of immunity; a defense against infection when there is no danger. It is an overreaction by the body's defense mechanisms to certain food, clothing, pollen, and other materials. The adrenal glands are important if an inflammation occurs because the body's defenses misconstrue certain materials. Because they also have endocrine functions aside from their reproductive functions, the reproductive glands are helpful in an allergic reaction. The hormones of the pituitary gland govern the other endocrine glands.

Hay Fever	Adrenal glands (p. 53) Reproductive glands (pp. 62-63) Pituitary (p. 41) Head / neck / sinus (pp. 43-46) Ileocecal valve (p. 55)	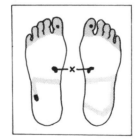 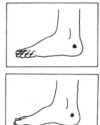

Hay fever is an allergic response of the upper respiratory tract, usually a response to pollen in the environment. Work head/neck/sinus and ileocecal valve (for mucus) reflex areas for additional help with this problem. Note the stress cue of sensitivity in the adrenal gland reflex area. Suggest a self-help technique applieed to the adrenal gland reflex area to help condition the body.

Infections

The guidelines utilized in reflex area selection include: reflex area influences (site of the infection) and function-related influences (adrenal glands, lymphatic glands, pituitary).

Sinusitis (See "Research")	Adrenal glands (p. 53) Head / neck / sinus (pp. 43-46) Ileocecal valve (p. 55) Pituitary (p. 41)	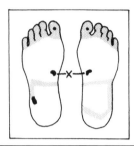

Sinuses are hollow cavities lined with thin membranes throughout the head region. Mucus coats these membranes to protect them. The only known anatomical function of the sinuses is to resonate the voice. The sinus cavities can become clogged with excessive mucus, causing headaches and congestion. When the cavities become infected, the condition is called sinusitis. All the toes need careful attention on all sides, as well as the tops and bottoms. The ileocecal valve is an important area for this problem. The valve is a passageway between the small and large intestines for control of the flow of wastes. The area around the ileocecal valve reflex area has a great deal of influence on the mucus level in the body. Work the adrenal gland reflex area for infection. Note the touch stress cues of hardening or thickening or sensitivity in the joints of the toes.

Sore Throat	Neck (p. 58) Adrenal glands (p. 53) Lymphatic glands (p. 61)	

Note the touch stress cues of thickening, hardening, or sensitivity in the tops, bottoms, and sides of the toes. Always work the adrenal gland reflex area for infections.

Tonsillitis	Neck (pp. 43-46) Lymphatic glands (p. 61) Adrenal glands (p. 53)	

Tonsillitis is an infection in the throat of the mass lymphoid tissue called the tonsils. Work the lymphatic reflex area, the neck reflex area, and the adrenal gland reflex area for infection. Search the bottom of the toe as the stem goes into the ball of the toe and work it thoroughly.

Lymphatic System

The guidelines utilized in reflex area selection include: reflex area influences (chest, spleen) and function-related influences (lymphatic glands, pituitary, thymus).

Breast	Chest (pp. 49-51) Lymphatic glands (p. 61) Pituitary (p. 41)	

The breasts can be considered part of the lymphatic system, as lymph nodes are spread throughout the breast area. The lymphatic nodes drain the fat portion of the milk during lactation. They are a vehicle for transferring infection to more distant parts. Plugged lymph nodes rather than malignancies are responsible for the majority of lumps detected. The pituitary reflex area is worked for any type of growth.

Note touch and sensitivity stress cues on the top of the foot.

Leukemia	Spleen (pp. 43-46) Lymphatic glands (p. 61) Thymus Liver (pp. 43-46)	

A chronic or acute disease characterized by the unrestrained growth of leukocytes, white blood cells. Symptoms include anemia and fatigue. Note the sensitivity stress cue in the spleen reflex area.

203

Musculo-Skeletal System Disorders

The guidelines utilized in reflex area selection include influences: reflex area (spine) and function-related (adrenal glands, solar plexus, thyroid, colon, kidneys, digestive system, endocrine system).

| **Arthritis** | Solar plexus (p. 47)
Kidneys (p. 51, p. 54)
Adrenal glands (p. 53)
Thyroid (p. 42)
Lymphatic drain (pp. 49-51) | 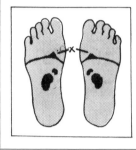 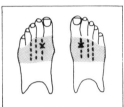 |

Arthritis is a general body condition coming from a variety of sources and generally associated with an inflammation of a joint. Because it is a general body condition, the whole foot should be worked. The kidneys can be useful in eliminating waste materials that can gather around the joints. The adrenal glands' inflammation-fighting qualities are important. According to recent studies, tension has an effect on arthritis. Working the solar plexus area for the relaxation of tension may help the root cause of arthritis. Note the visual stress cue of a bump on the tops of the feet, the kidney reflex areas.

| **Back Disorders** | Spine (pp. 57-59) | 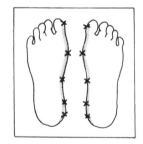  |

The spine is the support structure for the body and the housing structure for the spinal cord; the continuation of the brain below the skull. The spine (and its influence) go beyond its role as a supporting structure. The nerves originating from the spinal cord assert control over large segments of the torso and internal organs. The postural fatigue of the back can be a hidden nemesis in a myriad of problems, such as lung and digestive problems. Visual stress cues include: bunion, callousing, and lines on the sole of the foot radiating from the spine reflex areas.

Neck (Cervicals)	Neck (p. 58) Tops of shoulders (pp. 46-47) Solar plexus (p. 43)	

The seven cervicals of the neck are likely to be affected by tension and injuries, and their resulting problems are common. For cervical problems, work all sides of every toe, paying particular attention to the big toe. The cervicals are located on several lateral zones, with the seventh cervical encompassing the circular band at the base of the toe. The shoulder and solar plexus reflex areas should be worked in the appropriate areas on the feet because they, too, are areas commonly concerned with tension. Because nerves in the neck control the arm down to the fingertips, this area should be emphasized for numbness in the hands and for cold hands. This area provides should be emphasized for any head disorder, such as epilepsy, stroke, and brain injury. Visual stress cues include: curled toes, callousing, toes pressed together. Touch stress cues are located along the joints of the toes, especially the big toe.

Midback (Thoracics)	Spine (pp. 57-59) Solar plexus (p. 43)	

The vertebrae attached to the ribs are involved in upper back problems from the neck to the waistline. The spinal reflex area from the base of the big toe to the "waistline" on the foot should be worked. This area wraps around the inside of the foot. An accompanying reflex area for tension is the solar plexus. Make a press and assess observation to select target areas. Visual stress cues include: callousing along the inside of the foot, lines radiating from the spine reflex area. Touch stress cues includes sensitivity in the spine reflex areas.

Lower Back (Lumbars)	Spine (pp. 57-59) Hip (p. 59) Solar plexus (p. 43) Knee / leg (p. 60) Lymph / groin (p. 61)	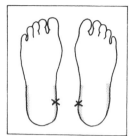 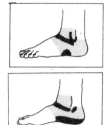 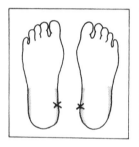 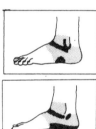

These five lumbar vertebrae bear much of the body's weight and therefore are subject to many problems. Work the area from the waistline into the hollow of the heel. The visual or touch stress cue of puffiness in the hollow can be indicative of lower back or bladder stress. These two reflex areas overlap. The lower back is interrelated with and can cause problems in many other areas. All reflex areas should be worked in conjunction with a problem in any one. Visual stress cues include: puffiness, callousing,

Lower Back / Tailbone	Spine (pp. 57-59) Lumbar vertebrae (p. 58)	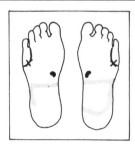 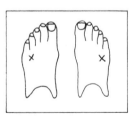

Rotation of the lower body and spine takes place in the lower back. The reflex area on the foot runs from the hollow of the heel down the inside edge of the heel. Helper reflex areas include areas on both the inside and outside of the heel extending into the ankle, the heel areas on the bottoms of the feet, and the lumbars. Make a press and assess observation to select target areas. Gauging tension in the ankle helps you assess tension in the lower back.

Bursitis	Shoulder (if affected) (pp. 48-50) Adrenal glands (p. 53) Colon (pp. 53-57)	

Bursitis is an inflammation of the bursa, a soft tissue sac that lies between body parts that move on each other (especially in joints). The shoulders are often susceptible to this problem. Working the adrenal glands areas on both feet can be helpful with the inflammation. Note the touch or visual stress cue of thickening or callousing in the shoulder reflex area.

Carpal tunnel syndrome	Heel of foot (pp. 53-57) Digestive system organs (pp. 53-57)	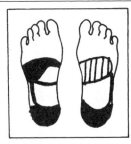

Carpal tunnel syndrome is a condition that results from compression of the median nerve at the wrist. The nerve is compressed within the carpal tunnel, a bony canal in the palm side of the wrist that provides passage for the median nerve to the hand. The irritation of the median nerve is specifically due to pressure from the transverse carpal ligament. Reflex area selection includes the heel of the foot which reflects the area of concern, the heel of the hand.

Gout	Kidneys (p. 53, p. 56) Corresponding body area	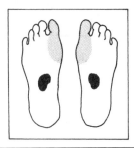

Gout is a hereditary metabolic disease and a form of acute arthritis. An excess of uric acid in the blood causes inflammation around a joint. Attacks are sudden and painful. The big toe is a frequent target for gout, but it is not the only area where it can occur. The kidneys control uric acid, and their reflex areas on the feet are therefore important. Note the touch stress cue of thickening or hardening in the kidney reflex area. Work the corresponding joint (referral area) in the hand as well. Be aware of the potential for sensitivity around the toe joint. Use light pressure. Be careful when applying desserts in the area.

Hernia	Lymphatic / groin (p. 61) Lower back (p. 58, p. 60) Hip (p. 59) Adrenal glands (p. 53)	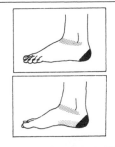 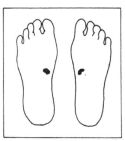

A hernia is a protrusion of an organ, most commonly the intestines, into another part of the body. For herniation of the groin apply technique to the lymphatic / groin reflex area. Also work the adrenal gland reflex area for muscle tone. Note the touch stress cues of thickening or hardening in the reflex area.

207

Hip Disorders	Hip / back / sciatic (p. 59) Lymphatic / groin (p. 61) Hip region (p. 60) Knee / leg (p. 60) Lower back (p. 58, p. 60)	

Hip problems have a variety of sources. The lower back is frequently the root cause of this problem. Search the hip region, the hip/back/sciatic, lymph/groin, and knee/leg for the stress cue of sensitivity in the reflex area. Note any protrusion of the bone on the outside of the foot (base of the fifth metatarsal). Take particular note of the stress cue if it is red and inflamed. Note the touch stress cue of thickened or hardened tonus in the hip reflex area.

Osteoporosis	Thyroid / Parathyroid (p. 42) Endocrine glands Liver (pp. 51-53) Digestive system (pp. 54-57)	

Osteoporosis is the thinning of the bones with reduction in bone mass due to depletion of calcium and bone protein. Osteoporosis predisposes a person to fractures, which are often slow to heal and heal poorly. It is more common in older adults, particularly post-menopausal women. Unchecked osteoporosis can lead to changes in posture, physical abnormality (particularly the form of hunched back known colloquially as "dowager's hump"), and decreased mobility. Osteoporosis can be detected by using tests that measure bone density. Calcium levels are regulated by the thyroid.

Sciatica	Hip / sciatic (p. 59) Lymphatic / groin (p. 61) Lower back / tailbone (p. 58, p. 60) Knee / leg (p. 60)	

Sciatica is a common term for a persistent pain around the sciatic nerve. The sciatic nerve is the largest nerve in the body. It branches from the lower back down both legs and branches again above the knee. From the knee it stirrups around the heel. The pain is a symptom. But the reason for most sciatic pain is pressure on a spinal nerve by a slipped disc. Direct pressure (i.e., from a poor seating position) is a less common cause for this pain. The hip/sciatic reflex area needs thorough coverage. Note the touch stress cue of thickening or hardening in the lymphatic/groin area and the top of the ankle bone where the hip/sciatic reflex area makes an upper loop. The lower back/tailbone reflex area and the bottom of the heel should be emphasized. Working the knee/leg reflex area can benefit this problem as well. Make a press and assess evaluation of the heel.

Shoulder Disorders	Shoulder (pp. 48-50) Neck (p. 58) Midback (p. 58) Arm (p. 54) Tops of the shoulders (pp. 46-47) Digestive system (pp. 54-57)	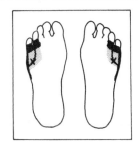

Pain in the shoulder can come from areas outside the shoulder region. The neck and midback region are helper reflex areas for this problem. Work the shoulder reflex areas on the tops and bottoms of the feet. The neck reflex areas should be thoroughly covered. Tenderness will frequently be encountered in the midback reflex area. The reflex areas of the arms and tops of the shoulders can provide additional help. Corns and callouses are frequently associated with this problem because of their ability to block the zone. Note the touch stress cues of thickening or sensitivity in the shoulder reflex area.

Whiplash	Neck (p. 58) Upper back (p. 58) Spine (pp. 57-59)	

Whiplash is a sprain of the muscles and tendons of the back of the neck caused by a sudden blow from the rear, such as occurs in an accident. Muscles and tendons throughout the neck and upper back are frequently involved. The first and second zones of the foot are of particular importance. Work the neck reflex area in all the toes. Cover the spine reflex area thoroughly. Work down the first and second zone between the big toe and the next toe in the lung reflex area. Note any stress cues in the toes and ball of the foot. Make a press and assess observation. Take note of the touch stress cue of thickening in the chest / lung reflex area on the top and bottom of the foot. Make a press and assess evaluation of the chest/lung reflex area on the bottom of the foot.

Neurological System

The guidelines utilized in reflex area selection include: reflex area influences (brain, brain stem, spine, tailbone) and function-related influences (kidneys, adrenal glands, pancreas, midback, eye/ear). Note the differences in parts of the toes (brain reflex areas) reflected in selection of reflex areas.

Alzheimer's (See "Research")	Brain (pp, 42-43) Brain stem (p. 59) Kidneys (p. 51, p. 54) Endocrine glands	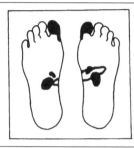

A progressive degenerative disease of the brain that leads to dementia. On a cellular level, Alzheimer is characterized by odd twisted filaments are called neurofibrillary tangles. On a functional level, there is degeneration of the cortical regions, especially the frontal and temporal lobes, of the brain.

Attention deficit disorder	Brain (pp. 43-46) Brain stem (p. 59) Adrenal glands (p. 53) Pancreas (pp. 52-53)	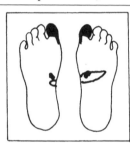

ADD (Attention Deficit Disorder): An inability to control behavior due to difficulty in processing neural stimuli.

Bell's palsy	Big toe (both sides) (pp. 42-45) Big toe below toe nail (p. 46) Endocrine glands	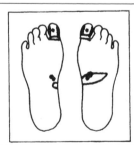

Paralysis of the facial nerve, the nerve that supplies the facial muscles on one side of the face. The cause of Bell's palsy is not known, but it is thought to be related to a virus (or to various viruses). Bell's palsy typically starts suddenly and causes paralysis of the muscles of the side of the face on which the facial nerve is affected. (The facial nerve is also known as the 7th cranial nerve). Note visual stress cue:of thickening of first joint of the big toe, reflecting the 7th cranial nerve.

Cerebral palsy (See "Research")	Brain (pp. 43-46) Top of head (p. 43)	

A syndrome of weakness, spasticity, poor coordination of the limbs and other muscles, impaired sensory perception, and sometimes impaired intelligence. The cause of cerebral palsy is not always known, although many cases are linked with lack of oxygen during birth. Treatment may include casting and braces to prevent further loss of limb function, speech therapy, physical therapy, occupational therapy, the use of augmentative communication devices, and the use of medications of botox injections to treat spasticity. Visual stress cues include: white speckling in the toes.

Epilepsy	Brain (pp. 43-46) Neck (p. 58) Eye / ear (pp. 46-47)	

When nerve cells in the brain fire electrical impulses at a rate of up to four times higher than normal, this causes a sort of electrical storm in the brain, known as a seizure. A pattern of repeated seizures is referred to as epilepsy. Known causes include head injuries, brain tumors, lead poisoning, maldevelopment of the brain, genetic and infectious illnesses. But in fully half of cases, no cause can be found. Medication controls seizures for the majority of patients.

Multiple sclerosis (See "Research")	Spine (pp. 57-59) Tailbone (p. 58)	

Symptoms of multiple sclerosis (MS) may range from numbness to paralysis and blindness. The progress, severity and specific symptoms cannot be foreseen. In medical terms, MS involves demyelinization of the white matter sometimes extending into the gray matter. Demyelinization is loss of myelin, the coating of nerve fibers that serves as insulation and permits efficient nerve fiber conduction. The "white matter" is the part of the brain which contains myelinated nerve fibers and appears white, whereas the gray matter is the cortex of the brain which contains nerve cell bodies and appears gray. When myelin is damaged in MS, nerve fiber conduction is faulty or absent. Impaired bodily functions or altered sensations associated with those demyelinated nerve fibers give rise to the symptoms of MS. Note stress cues in the tailbone reflex area.

| **Numbness in the Fingertips** | Seventh cervical (p. 42) Solar plexus (p. 47) Midback (p. 58) | |

The seventh cervical can affect everything from the base of the neck down into the fingertips. The cervical vertebrae are vulnerable to tension. Tension in the solar plexus area can lead to tension in the neck. Concentrate on the seventh cervical and the solar plexus reflex areas of the feet. Tension in the midback can contribute to problems. Note the touch stress cue of hardening in the seventh cervical reflex area.

| **Paralysis** | Eye / ear (pp. 46-47) Entire body of the foot Neck (p. 58) Spine (pp. 57-59) Top of head (p. 43) | |

Paralysis is the loss of voluntary movement resulting from the failure of nerve impulses to reach voluntary muscles. It has many causes (i.e., stroke, injury, etc.). Paralysis requires extreme dedication because of a variety of factors: the victim's age, the length of time since the injury, and the extent of the damage – all of which influence the outcome of work. Note the touch stress cue of thickening or hardening in the neck reflex area, the eye / ear reflex area, and the base of the toes.

| **Parkinson's disease** | Cerebellum (esp. left side) (p. 44) Neck (side of toe) (p. 44) | |

An abnormal condition of the nervous system caused by degeneration of an area of the brain called the basal ganglia and by low production of the neurotransmitter dopamine. The disease results in rigidity of the muscles, slow body movement and tremor. Note touch stress cues includes: hard tonus on the lateral (outside) at the first joint and below, reflecting the cerebellum reflex area.

Stroke Brain Injury	Top of head (p. 43) Head (pp. 43-46) Eye / ear (pp. 46-47) Solar plexus (p. 47) Spine (pp. 57-59)	

A stroke is a sudden rupture or clotting of a blood vessel in the brain. Work the top of the head reflex area on the big toe opposite the side of the stroke. Work the tops of the smaller toes also. Technique should be applieed to the head and spine reflex areas.

Psychological Disorders

Anxiety	Solar plexus (p. 47) Endocrine glands Pancreas (pp. 51-53)	

A feeling of apprehension, worry, uneasiness or dread especially of the future. Note stress cues including: sensitivity in the adrenal gland reflex areas and touch stress cues of thickening in the solar plexus reflex area.

Depression	Endocrine glands Solar plexus (p. 47) Pancreas (pp. 51-53) Head (pp. 43-46)	

The factors contributing to depression can be psychological or physical. Among physical factors are the endocrine glands and their effects on the vigor and degree of activity. Another factor can be tension as a potential source of depression or as a complicating element. Blood sugar levels have been suspected in mood fluctuations. The pancreas is involved in controlling the blood sugar level with insulin. Note the touch stress cue of thickened or hardened tonus in the pancreas reflex area. Consider the flexibility of the toes.

Reproductive System

The guidelines utilized in reflex area selection include: reflex area influences (uterus, ovaries, fallopian tubes, prostate, testicles,) and function-related influences (solar plexus, pituitary, endocrine glands, lower back, bladder).

Birthing / Pregnancy	Solar plexus (p. 47) Reproductive glands (pp. 62-63) Pituitary (p. 41) Endocrine glands Lower back / Bladder (p. 58)	

Pregnancy and birthing are the condition of carrying a developing embryo to term as a child. Reflexology work throughout the pregnancy has been shown to ease pregnancy and facilitate the birthing process. Technique is applied to the solar plexus reflex area to ease tension. Caution: Reflexology work is a stressor. It is a positive stressor, however, care should be taken not to apply take heavy pressure or for too long a time period.

Impotence	Reproductive glands (pp. 62-63) Lower back (p. 58) Bladder (p. 58)	

Impotence or erectile dysfunction is the consistent inability to sustain an erection sufficient for sexual intercourse, inability to achieve ejaculation, or both. Impotence can be a total inability to achieve erection or ejaculation, an inconsistent ability to do so, or a tendency to sustain only brief erections. Impotence usually has a physical cause, such as disease, injury, drug side-effects, or a disorder that impairs blood flow in the penis. Impotence can also have an emotional cause.

Infertility	Male: Testes (pp. 62-63) Prostate (pp. 62-63) Lymphatic / groin (p. 61) Female: Uterus (pp. 62-63) Ovaries (pp. 62-63) Fallopian tube (p. 61)	

Infertility is the inability to conceive a child because of structural, endocrine gland, or psychological problems. Both partners are to be considered, unless a professional diagnosis has already pointed to one partner as the source of the problem.

For women, a number of malfunctions of the egg-producing mechanism and transport system can occur. The fallopian tubes may be blocked, for example. In some cases working the pituitary area on each big toe has proven beneficial in normalizing the monthly ovulation cycle. At times emotions are a factor. Expectation and worry may contribute to the overall imbalances in the systems. The solar plexus reflex area needs emphasis. Another possibility is that the male may not be producing enough sperm to cause conception. Thus the testicle and prostate reflex areas need emphasis. The rest of the endocrine gland reflex areas are interrelated with the reproductive functions. Work them thoroughly for any reproductive dysfunction. Note any stress cues of thick or hardened tonus in the lymphatic / groin reflex area.

Menstruation / Menopause (See "Research")	Uterus (pp. 62-63) Ovary (pp. 62-63) Fallopian tubes (p. 61) Lower back (p. 58)	

The female reproductive areas include the uterus, the ovaries, and the fallopian tubes which join them. These areas are commonly affected by menstrual problems, menopause, and infertility. Reflex areas to emphasize on the feet include all of the reproductive reflex areas and the endocrine gland reflex areas because of the interrelationship of all the glands. Note the touch stress cues of thickening and sensitivity in the reproductive reflex areas.

For menstrual problems and menopausal discomfort, work of the above areas are important, with special emphasis on the uterus reflex area. Infertility can be caused by infection, blocked fallopian tube, endocrine gland dysfunction, or psychological problems. Thus all of the reproductive reflex areas and the other endocrine gland reflex areas are important ones to emphasize. A hysterectomy is the surgical removal of the uterus. Scar tissue and adhesions may be reflected as the touch stress cues of thickening or hardening.

Post-partum depression	Brain stem (p. 59) Endocrine system Solar plexus (p. 47) Lymphatic system (p. 61)	

Depression that occurs in about 3% of women following birth with feelings of inadequacy, hopelessness, inability to cope, tearfulness, mood swings, fatigue, insomnia. Reflex areas are selected on the basis of function: regulation of hormones, relaxation and elimination.

Premenstrual syndrome (See "Research")	Uterus (pp. 62-63) Ovaries (pp. 62-63) Solar plexus (p. 47) Groin / lymphatic glands (p. 61)	

A combination of physical and mood disturbances that occur after ovulation and normally end with the onset of the menstrual flow. Premenstrual syndrome (PMS) is believed to be a disorder of the neurotransmitters and other hormones. In its most severe form, it can be truly disabling for part of the month, and strongly resembles a type of bipolar disorder. Reflex areas are selected on the basis of function, the regulation of hormones.

Prostate Disorders	Prostate (pp. 62-63) Testicle (pp. 62-63) Lymphatic glands / groin (p. 61) Lower back / bladder (p. 58)	

The prostate is a male gland behind the outlet of the bladder surrounding the urethra. It contributes the thin, milky alkaline fluid to the semen. The prostate will enlarge due to disease or injury, causing the continued urge to urinate with some discomfort. This is common in middle-aged to older men.

Work the prostate/uterus reflex area on the feet. The rest of the reproductive and lower back reflex areas should be worked. Check flexibility of the ankle with the Ankle Rotation Technique. Note the touch stress cues of thickening and hardening.

Respiratory System

The guidelines utilized in reflex area selection include: reflex area influences (lungs, diaphragm) and function-related influences (adrenal glands, solar plexus, ileocecal valve, colon).

Asthma (See "Research")	Adrenal glands (p. 53) Ileocecal valve (p. 56) Solar plexus (p. 47) Lungs (pp. 48-50)	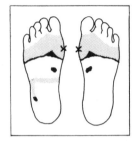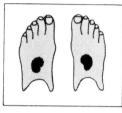

Asthma is an allergic condition associated with wheezing, coughing, and difficulty in exhaling. Adrenaline is administered by a doctor for asthma episodes. The adrenal glands produce their own adrenaline, so this area on the feet is emphasized for asthma. The ileocecal valve reflex area is worked for the control of mucus. Working the solar plexus reflex area eases the tension that often accompanies asthma. Note the visual, press and assess and sensitivity stress cues in the ball of the foot.

Bronchitis	Chest / lung (pp. 48-50) Adrenal glands (p. 53)	

Chronic bronchitis usually is defined clinically as a daily cough with production of sputum for 3 months, two years in a row. In chronic bronchitis, there is inflammation and swelling of the lining of the airways that lead to narrowing and obstruction of the airways. The inflammation stimulates production of mucous (sputum), which can cause further obstruction of the airways. Obstruction of the airways, especially with mucus, increases the likelihood of bacterial lung infections. The adrenal gland reflex area is worked for its anti-inflammation qualities. Note the visual, press and assess and sensitivity stress cues in the ball of the foot.

Emphysema	Lung (pp. 48-50) Ileocecal (p. 56) Solar plexus (p. 47) Colon (pp. 54-57)	

Emphysema is a lung condition in which exhaling is difficult. The lung sac becomes inelastic. Tension is also a major contributor to this problem. Excess mucus aggravates the situation even further. Cover the lung reflex areas on the feet thoroughly. Also emphasize the ileocecal valve reflex area for mucus and the solar plexus reflex area for tension. Note the stress cues in the ball of the foot. Make a press and assess observation to select target areas for technique application emphasis.

Skin Disorders

The guidelines utilized in reflex area selection include: function-related influences (adrenal glands, reproductive glands, kidneys, thyroid, adrenal glands, pituitary, lymphatic glands, solar plexus, spine). The skin is viewed as the largest organ of the body thus the number of functionally-related reflex areas.

Sjkin Disorders	Reproductive glands (pp. 62-63) Kidneys (p. 51, p. 54) Thyroid (p. 42) Adrenal glands (p. 53) Pituitary (p. 41)	

The skin is considered an organ. Its disorders are visible and thus attract more attention than those of a similar magnitude affecting other organs. The skin is one of the body's eliminators. Improper elimination can blemish the skin. The functioning of the kidneys and endocrine glands is important. Areas of emphasis depend on the type of disorder. Acne requires emphasis of the reproductive and the pituitary reflex areas. Dry skin or oily skin involves the thyroid and pituitary reflex areas.

Eczema	Endocrine glands Solar plexus (p. 47) Kidneys (p. 51, p. 54) Lymphatic glands (p. 61)	

Eczema is a disorder involving dryness of skin. The thyroid and adrenal gland reflex areas have often been found to be helpful with this disorder. The skin contributes to the waste elimination process. Working the lymphatic and kidney reflex areas helps the problem by easing some of this burden. Note any visual or touch stress cues in the kidney reflex area on the top and bottom of the foot.

| Psoriasis | Kidneys (p. 51, p. 54)
Thyroid (p. 42)
Adrenal glands (p. 53)
Pituitary (p. 41) | |

Psoriasis is a disorder of the outer layer of skin. It typically looks like thickened red blotches with a scale surface, mostly affecting the scalp, back, and arms. In normal skin, old cells form the outer layer of skin and new cells are formed underneath. In psoriasis, the situation is accelerated, with new cells being formed before the old cells can be shed. The endocrine glands, particularly the thyroid and adrenal glands, contribute to this process. The kidneys, as chief eliminators of the body, take some of the burden off the skin (which also eliminates waste products).

| Shingles | Spine (dermatome level appropriate to rash) (pp. 57-59) | |

An acute infection caused by the virus Herpes zoster, which also causes chicken pox. Shingles usually emerges in adulthood after exposure to chicken pox or reactivation of the chicken pox virus, which can remain latent in body tissues for years until the immune system is weakened. It is an extraordinarily painful condition that involves inflammation of sensory nerves. The outbreak of rash occurs along a segment or segments of the dermatomes that branch off the spinal cord. The spinal reflex area relative to the rash is selected for technique emphasis. See p. 11 for dermatome chart.

Urinary System

The guidelines utilized in reflex area selection include: reflex area influences (bladder, kidney, ureter tubes) and function-related influences (adrenal glands, lymphatic glands).

| Bladder Infection / Urinary infection | Bladder (p. 56)
Kidney (p. 51, p. 54)
Ureter tubes (pp. 57-58)
Adrenal glands (p. 53) | |

The bladder is the reservoir for holding urine. The bladder/lower back reflex areas overlap and are located in the hollow of the heel. (See Lower Back.) The visual or touch stress cue of puffiness here may indicate stress in the bladder or lower back. Note stress cues in other urinary system reflex areas, the kidneys, and ureter tubes. Make a press and assess observation of the reflex area to note target areas.

Incontinence	Brain stem (p. 59) Bladder (p. 56) Kidney (p. 51, p. 54) Ureter tubes (pp. 57-58)	

The bladder is the reservoir for holding urine. The brain stem is involved in metabolic control over basic functions including continence. The bladder/lower back reflex areas overlap and are located in the hollow of the heel. (See Lower Back.) The visual or touch stress cue of puffiness here may indicate stress in the bladder or lower back. Note stress cues in the brain stem reflex area as well as the reflex areas of the urinary system, the kidneys and ureter tubes. Make a press and assess observation of the reflex areas to note target areas.

Kidney infection	Kidney (p. 51, p. 54) Ureter tubes (p. 56) Bladder (pp. 57-58) Adrenal glands (p. 53)	

The most common kidney disorders involve the kidneys' filtration function. The nephrons, or little filters (of which there are about a million in the kidneys), can become infected. The flow of urine can be obstructed. The ureter tubes can be blocked by stones, pressure from other organs, and enlargement of the prostate (in men). The urine can become stagnated and can carry infection, which may lead to serious damage. The kidneys can be damaged by hypertension. (See Hypertension.) Edema or excessive accumulation of fluids in the body is at times caused by kidney disease. Many conditions can cause edema. The kidney reflex areas, however, should always be worked to eliminate this excess. Toxicity in the body can be assisted by working the kidney reflex area. The toxins are a by-product of cell metabolism. The kidneys, as chief eliminators can filter the blood, disposing of the waste. Concentrate work on the entire second zone. Note the touch stress cue of thickening or hardening in the kidney reflex area.

Kidney Stones (See "Research")	Kidneys (p. 51, p. 54) Ureter tubes (p. 56) Bladder (pp. 57-58)	

Kidney stones occur when the urine is too concentrated. Various substances, such as calcium salts, uric acid, and other materials crystallize. They can pass out without notice when they are small. However, if they become large, the sensitive ureter tubes can be affected. The ureters are elastic, but as the large kidney stones try to pass out, their jagged edges catch on the narrow sensitive walls. Surgery may become necessary to remove them. Whatever the situation, the kidneys, ureters, and bladder reflex areas on the feet need careful attention. Concentrate on the entire second zone. Note any stress cues in the second toe. Note any toe that crosses over another toe.

Miscellaneous

Anemia	Spleen (pp. 52-53) Liver (p. 51-53) Thymus Lymphatic glands (p. 61)	

Anemia, a lack of iron in the blood cells, is a symptom of many diseases. The spleen, as a recycler of iron, is important in the manufacture of hemoglobin. Hemoglobin is an iron-containing protein in the red blood cells that is responsible for carrying oxygen from the lungs to the body tissues. The liver and spleen overlap in some functions.

Chronic fatigue syndrome	Pancreas (pp. 51-53) Kidneys (p. 51, p. 54) Brain stem (p. 59) Liver (p. 51-53)	

A debilitating medical condition, chronic in nature, cause unknown, diagnosis by exclusion, no known verified test, treatment by relief of symptoms, life style changes, and occasionally time. There has been some debate over the existence and causes of this condition but speculation includes virus infection or other transient traumatic condition, stress and toxins. Selected reflex areas include those of the pancreas (energy), kidneys (elimination), brain stem (regulation of metabolism), and liver for elimination of toxins.

Dizziness (Vertigo)	Eye / ear (pp. 46-47) Solar plexus (p. 47)	

The causes of dizziness are varied. A common cause is an infection of the inner ear, which contains the mechanism for balance. Vertigo describes a condition in which the room seems to be spinning. Note the touch stress cue of thickening in the eye/ear reflex area, particularly between the second and third toes. If dizziness is chronic, apply technique to all of the toes, the ball of the foot, and the outside of the big toe.

Environmental sensitivity	Adrenal glands (p. 53) Mid spine (pp. 58-59) Pancreas (p. 51, p. 54) Kidneys (p. 51, p. 54) Lymphatic glands (p. 61) Liver (pp. 51-53)	

Environmental sensitivity is a "chronic, recurring disease caused by a person's inability to tolerate an environmental chemical or class of foreign chemicals" resulting in symptoms including those that resemble allergic reactions, general malaise, or effecting specific organs such as the lungs.

Fainting	Pituitary (p. 32)	

Fainting is caused by sudden insufficient blood supply to the brain. The pituitary reflex area of both big toes are considered revival points. Apply the *thumb hook and back up* technique repeatedly to the pituitary reflex area. Also work the adrenal gland reflex area. Helper areas include the eye/ear, solar plexus, pituitary, and adrenal gland reflex areas.

Fever	Pituitary (p. 32)	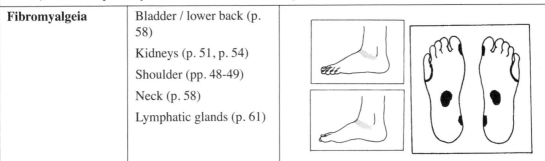

A fever is an increase in body temperature associated with infection (also a symptom of other illnesses). Work the pituitary reflex area and the adrenal gland reflex areas.

Fibromyalgeia	Bladder / lower back (p. 58) Kidneys (p. 51, p. 54) Shoulder (pp. 48-49) Neck (p. 58) Lymphatic glands (p. 61)	

Also known as fibrositis, fibromyalgeia chronically causes pain, stiffness, and tenderness of muscles, tendons, and joints without detectable inflammation. Fibromyalgeia does not cause body damage or deformity. However, undue fatigue plagues 90% of patients with fibromyalgeia. Sleep disorder is common in patients with fibromyalgeia. Fibromyalgeia can be associated with other rheumatic conditions. Irritable bowel syndrome can occur with fibromyalgeia. There is no test for the diagnosis of fibromyalgeia.

Headaches, **Migraine headache** (See "Research")	Head / neck / sinus (pp. 41-45) Solar plexus (p. 47) Tailbone and spine (p. 58)	

Headaches occur in response to certain drugs, physical conditions, and stress. The toes represent the head and neck area. The big toe in itself is a study for tension in the head and neck. Try working all through the head and neck reflex areas on the feet. The solar plexus reflex area needs attention for reducing tension.Try the Side to Side Dessert Technique to lessen the tension associated with a migraine. Migraine is a common and particularly distressing type of headache. Migraines are not yet fully understood. The areas mentioned above are important. The spine reflex area also needs careful attention along its entire length, particularly the tailbone reflex area. Unusual as this sounds, many migraines have been linked to injuries in this area. Note the results of a press and assess evaluation of the big toe.

Insomnia	Solar plexus (p. 47) Adrenal glands (p. 53) Brain stem (p. 59)	

A complaint that an individual has trouble falling asleep or staying asleep long enough to feel rested. Causes include sleep apnea (interruption in oxygen), periodic limb movements, response to allergies (congestion and swelling contribute to apnea) and narcolepsy. Some 45% of insomnia is attributed to anxiety.

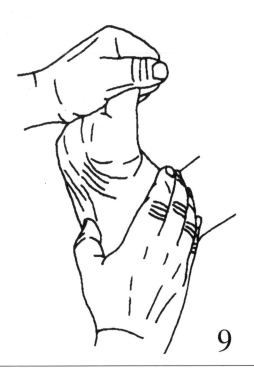

9

The Complete Reflexologist

The Complete Reflexologist

The skills you have acquired thus far provide the basis for the services you will furnish to your clientele. Ultimately, it is your ability to communicate your work that will be of value to your client, other professionals and those who pay for expert services such as insurers. Further, your knowledge of stress patterns and protocols to address them will be of value to establish reflexology use in evidence-based medicine. As a complete reflexologist you will, thus, project the attitude of a professional and expert in a unique and valued field.

This chapter features how to improve your skills through improving your communication abilities. To provide some perspective for putting together observation, assessment and communication, examples of interactions with clients follow. Also included are how to use visual feedback to demonstrate your skills and noting stress patterns to further your professional knowledge.

This chapter also includes how to recognize a stress pattern with an inference of a stress-related disorder. Just as stress researcher Hans Selye studied stereotypical responses to stress, the complete reflexologist notes patterns of stress cues in the feet. As you become more and more proficient at assessing the feet, you will notice whole foot patterns of stress cues. Making a study of the wear and tear patterns makes you a participant in the broader picture of the profession and a contributor to the field of knowledge.

You will note the use of photographs, taken here with a digital camera. Use of a digital or Polaroid camera makes instantly available to the client a glimpse of the stress cues of his or her feet. Take a picture before and after a session and over the course of your work. Your observations and work are made visual and value is, thus, added to your service. In addition, photos can record and document your work for communication with other reflexologists and medical professionals as well as in cases of workman's compensation or insurance reimbursement.

Developing Communication Skills

Becoming a skilled observer provides focus for your work and an opportunity to communicate with your client. Communicating observations and inferences creates client confidence in your credibility.

The following photos provide you the opportunity to observe a variety of feet. With skills honed by comparing and contrasting feet - the left foot to right foot, the feet of this individual to the feet of another - you build assurance in your work. The comments illustrate, in an abbreviated form, how to communicate your skill as a practitioner to the client, specifically: (1) use of stress cue observations and inferences, (2) how stress cues can demonstrate the value of your services to the client (see "Evaluating Body Stress Inferences") and (3) how to document and/or demonstrate the efficacy of your work (see "Observing and Noting Changes in the Stress Response" and "Planning").

Communication of Assessment

Observing stress cues and drawing inferences form a frame work for your work. Communicating your assessment includes: noting the stress cue observations as you find them, asking a question (foot stress inference) appropriate to the location and patterns of the stress cue (reflex stress inference) to see if the individual perceives as a problem the stress or stress pattern that you have observed (body stress inference). Comments to the client are a part of the process of planning future work.

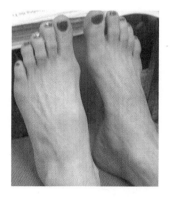

Stress cue observation: Taut tendons; curled, knobby toes pressed together; longer second toes; bumps and bulges; bumps on top of the foot.
Foot stress inference: Exhaustion stage (50-something female)
Reflex stress inference: Overall musculo-skeletal reflex areas; gallbladder, kidney and pancreas reflex areas
Body stress inference questions: Does your neck bother you? Does your chest or upper back bother you? Does your hip bother you? Do you have digestive problems?
Body stress response: Yes, I have problems throughout my muscles and joints as well as gallbladder problems.
Comments to client: I see quite a few stress cues that have been here for a while. These are stress cues, not necessarily disorders, but there does seem to be quite a bit of stress in the musculo-skeletal system. That seems to match your answers to observations about the stress cues. It will take some time to reach goals but you can speed it up with self-help.

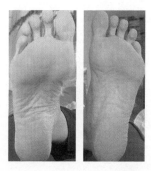

Stress cues: Longer second toe (one foot), extreme curled toe/wear spot, callousing, tailor's bunion, high arch, lined arch, callousing around heel, two extremely different feet.
Foot stress inference: Adaptive stage of adaptation
Reflex stress inference: Upper back stress, mid-back stress, lower back stress, hips, ear reflex area
Body stress inference: Do you have ringing in the ears? Does your hearing

bother you? Does your upper back bother you? Does your lower back bother you? Do your hips bother you?

Body stress response: Yes to all.

Comments to client: When I noted that one foot does not match the other, you noted that one leg is shorter. Client: why are the two feet different? Basically, it has to do the fact that because of accident, injury and other factors we tend to put more weight, more stress on one foot versus the other. Because the weight-bearing is so much on one side, I usually ask, How are your hips?

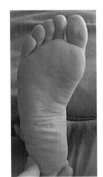

Stress cues: Lined arch, high arch, toes pressed together

Foot stress inference: Alarm stage of adaptation

Reflex stress inference: Neck, shoulder, mid-back, and pituitary reflex areas

Body stress inference: Does your neck bother you? Does your upper back bother you? Does your mid-back bother you? Have you injured your back? Do you have headaches? Fatigue?

Body stress response: Yes to all.

Comments to client: (The stress cues seen here are more than expected in a seventeen year old's feet. Trying to understand why, I asked about injury. The answer was, Yes, a car accident.) There are a fair amount of stress cues, but at your age it's easier to work with before they become set.

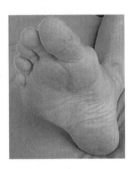

Stress cues: Callousing, bunion, high arch curled and pressed toes, lined arch

Foot stress inference: Adaptive stage of adaptation

Reflex stress inference: Ear, upper back, neck reflex areas

Body stress inferences: Does your back bother you? Do your ears bother you?

Body stress response: No to everything except for thyroid problem.

Comments to client: If you're not experiencing any problems, it might be a good idea to work on these areas before they become problems. (This will not be an easy client. She does not have a real awareness of what's going on with her body. Any changes that occur due to reflexology work, may not be noticed. And, since the changes will take a fair amount of work, she may not have the patience to seek sufficient sessions.)

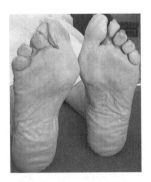

Stress cues: Feet do not match; extreme bunion, extreme curled and pressed toes, thick toenails, mottled color

Foot stress inferences: Exhaustion stage of adaptation (84 year-old woman)

Reflex stress inferences: Head, ear, chest reflex areas

Body stress inferences: Do you have hearing problems? Do you have problems in the chest? How's your memory? Do you have circulation problems?

Body stress response: Yes to all.

Comments to client: There are quite a few stress cues here that have been here for a while. It will take a fair amount of work to lessen the stress patterns in the chest, lung, upper back and neck reflex areas. Consistent self-help will help.

S. O. A. P. P. Formula Assessment

Assessments as those noted above can be expanded and utilized in a S. O. A. P. P. form. Presented here is an example.

Subjective: Terri, a forty-something single mother of two, felt her body was over-stressed and out-of-whack. She is self-employed in a standing profession, spending long hours on her feet. Her feet felt numb at times. She described stress in her personal life as well as digestive complaints, high blood pressure, and a perception that a rib was out of place.

Objective: Observing the visual stress cues on her feet, I saw an overall, general pattern of stress: feet that do not match, toes pressed together, callousing on the big toe, bulge on the big toe of left foot, curled and retracted third toe on the left foot, callousing on the ball of the foot, tailor's bunions, lined high arch, and callousing around the heel. Touch stress cues included an abundance of thick areas with some hardened tonus. There was an overall tightness about the foot. Initially there was no sensitivity, but over time, sensitivity appeared.

Assessment: From these stress cue observations, I drew the (foot stress) inference that the stress cues in her feet showed an adaptive stage of adaptation with some verging on exhaustion. The (reflex stress) inference is that is the level of stress is appropriate to her age and occupation with some over stressing. The further (body stress) inference is that an overall pattern of stress existed.

Plan: The client's goals can be met by addressing foot pain and overall stress with sessions scheduled once a week for two to three months.

Result: Terri has been using my reflexology services weekly for several years now. Her use of reflexology evolved over time from initial general stress reduction to addressing what she perceives as her weakest links. Early on, she dropped the weekly services of her chiropractor and her acupuncturist in preference for reflexology services. Her biggest revelation is that the physical stress cues were linked to her emotional responses.

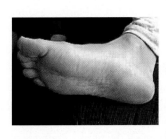
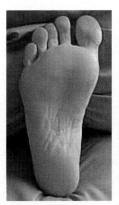
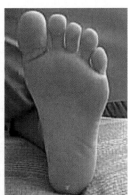
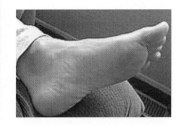

Using Visual Feedback

Photographing a stress cue, a foot or both feet provides visual feedback to the client. Alternatively, showing the client a stress cue or describing it can give him or her a sense of what you're assessing in the feet. For some clients, seeing the photograph or stress cue provides a confirmation about his or her health perceptions. For others, it demonstrates that there's something there and confers validity on your work.

The client whose feet are pictured in photos **1** and **1a** complained of breathing problems that she attributed to environmental sensitivity resulting from exposure to hair sprays and other chemicals during years of work as a cosmetologist. Press and assess stress cue observation showed white sheets in the lung reflex areas. While the client was shocked to see the photos of her feet, they provided confirmation of long-held feelings that her system had been "attacked" by environmental factors. Over time, the white sheeting diminished in size and gradually faded out. She has been a client for a number of years and we've moved on to other health goals.

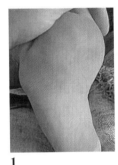 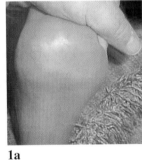 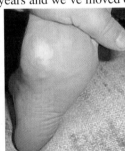 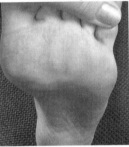

1   **1a**   **2**   **3**

Compare and contrast the stress cues of the feet pictured above. Such comparisons provide an opportunity to sharpen your knowledge base of reflex areas for future work. The twenty-something client whose foot is pictured in photo **2** knew she had a hiatal hernia problem but the sight of the stress cue gave her the sense that there was something real going on with her body. The woman whose feet are pictured in photo **3** was under doctor's care and took medication for severe and debilitating asthma attacks.

Photographing Before and After Work

Photographing stress cues helps you build a library for future reference and/or professional presentations. In addition, it gives you a "before" photo so that you can demonstrate later to the client the physical effects of your work. Taking a picture before and after your work demonstrates that you've effectively created change and worked toward meeting your client's goal.

Photos can be taken before and after a single session. You, thus, demonstrate visually to the client the impact of your work. For example, in the photos to the right, note the improved overall color of the feet before the session (pictured above) and after the session (pictured below). Photos taken at the commencement of your sessions and periodically throughout a series of sessions show the impact of your work. Some changes may be subtle but some will be dramatic.

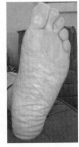

Studying Stress Patterns

As noted in the previous section, stress cues show specific stereotypical responses to stress that are related to specific parts of the body. For example, the curled little toe resting on the base of the toes can show stress in the ear reflex area. Moreover, the partially curled little toe may signal ringing in the ears while the fully curled toe may indicate hearing problems. Such observations will add to your depth as a skilled practitioner.

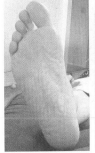
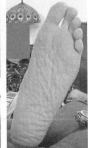

George Leger of Winnipeg, for example, observed the feet of the individuals in his father's Alzheimer's ward. He noted the same stress cue in 18 of the 20 pairs of feet: a bulge in the big toe that created a flap extending to the second and third toes at times. Ruth Hahn of Piqua, Ohio who directed the Rehabilitation Center for Neurological Development and applied reflexology to brain injured individuals noted that the brain injured have "pointy" toes. While such observations have not been scientifically validated, they open the door to a new area of reflexology study: identifying stereotypical patterns of stress cues to aid in the assessment and treatment of conditions.

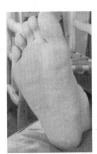
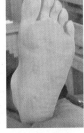

Stress cues can form a pattern occupying whole parts of the foot. In the following examples you will see how stress-related disorders, age, heredity, occupation, and all the other factors of stress history can play a role in a stress pattern as reflected in the feet.

Occupation Related Stress Pattern

The over-worked feet pictured to the right reflect the stress cue patterns common to those in standing occupations: flat feet that have spread, excessive color in one instance, lined arch in another, and mottled color in another.

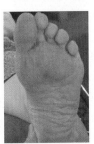
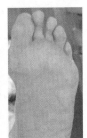

231

Stress-Related Disorder Patterns

Whole parts of the foot can show the stress cue pattern of a stress-related disorder. The stress cues pictured in the foot to the left is typical of a lower back pattern of stress. The extreme ankle puffiness in the hip reflex area and the mottled color showing impingement of circulation to the lower back and consequently to feet. The bunion and pressed toes reflect further musculo-skeletal reflex areas under stress.

The side views of the feet pictured below also show traits common to a lower back pattern of stress. Note the high arches, the epi-center of the lines in the arch radiating from the low back reflex areas, the bumps on the inside of the foot, and S-shape of the spine reflex area.

The feet pictured below (**A**) are those of a forty-year old male in a stressful profession with concerns about high levels of tension and heart palpitations. The other feet pictured below (**B**) are those of an eighty-year male old with congestive heart failure and musculo-skeletal problems. The photos show similar stress cue features: very high arch; curled, pressed and retracted toes; heavy pressure on the balls of the feet; and a bump on top of the foot. "Heart feet" was the comment of the dean of a nursing school familiar with our work when viewing similar feet. Possibilities of work with the older man are different from those of the younger. Work with the older man resulted in lessened swelling of the feet, easier breathing, and leveling of an erratic heart beat as measured by a heart monitor. Following reflexology work, the younger man experienced a general feeling of relaxation.

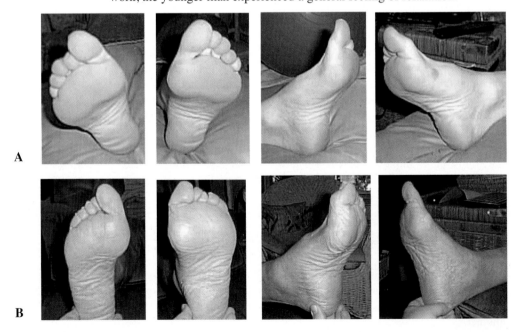

A

B

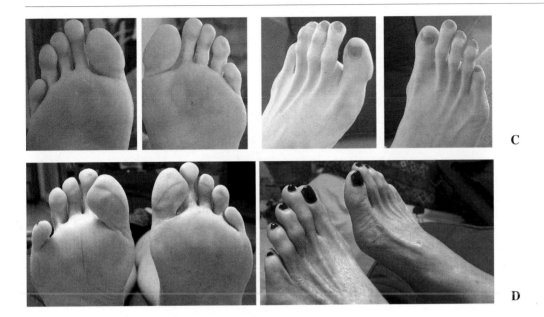

C

D

Foot Structure Stress Patterns

The structure of the foot reflects the musculo-skeletal system. Stress cues of the structure of the foot, thus, reflect a musculo-skeletal stress pattern. Bunions, for example, frequently reflect stress in the chest and upper back. Pictured above, the feet of a daughter and mother illustrate an extreme structural foot stress pattern as well as age appropriateness and the role of heredity.

The feet of the thirty-something daughter (C) show significant stress cues (longer second, third and fourth toes) as do the feet of her seventy-something mother (D). Additional structural stress cues include calloused big toe, bunions, tailor's bunions, knobby toes, taut tendons, and curled little toes with wear spots. Both reported a musculo-skeletal stress pattern: tension in the upper back, chest, and neck. Stress cues in the mother's feet include bulges in the big toes. She reported no loss of memory but a mother with Alzheimer's. While both pairs of feet show significant stress cues, the mother's stress cues are more age appropriate. The accelerated rate of the daughter's stress cues is perhaps attributable to stress history, stressed habits, stressed home or workplace, and/or abilities to handle stress.

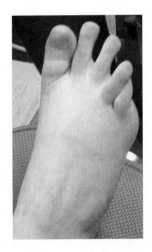

In contrast to the heredity factors pictured above, the foot photo to the right shows a foot structure stress pattern resulting from whiplash suffered in a car accident. The owner of this foot reported neck, upper back, and shoe-buying problems. She could not make her toes move together.

233

Foot Reflexology Charts

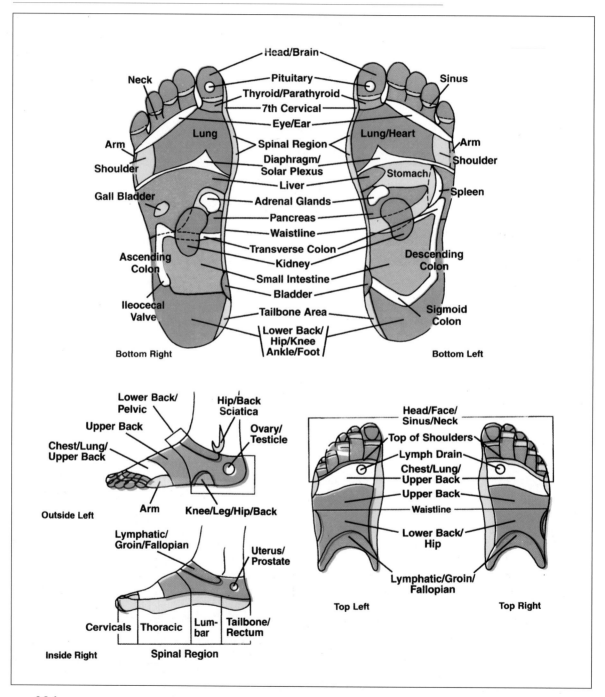